**Heidelberg
Science
Library**

Volume

10

Heidelberg
Science
Library

Walter Fuhrmann
Friedrich Vogel

translated by Sabine Kurth

Genetic
Counseling

Second Edition

Springer-Verlag
New York
Heidelberg
Berlin
1976

Walter Fuhrmann
Institut für Humangenetik
Giessen, West Germany

Friedrich Vogel
Institut für Anthropologie und Humangenetik
Heidelberg, West Germany

Library of Congress Cataloging in Publication Data

Fuhrmann, Walter, 1924–
  Genetic counseling.
  (Heidelberg science library; 10)
  Translation of Genetische Familienberatung.
  Bibliography: p. 129
  Includes index.
  1. Genetic counseling. I. Vogel, Friedrich, 1925–   joint author.
II. Title. III. Series. [DNLM: 1. Genetic counseling. 2. Hereditary
diseases. QZ50 F959g]
RB155.F813   1975   616'.042   75-28155

Printed in the United States of America

ISBN 0-387-90151-5   Springer-Verlag   New York

ISBN 3-540-90151-5   Springer-Verlag   Berlin   Heidelberg

Preface to the
Second Edition

In the second edition a new chapter on the prenatal diagnosis of genetic anomalies has been added. The discussion
has been deliberately limited to such aspects as are important to the practicing physician, especially the indications for such testing. The methods themselves are highly
specialized, as are the test facilities. The practicing physician cannot apply them himself in any case. We also added
passages concerning counseling criteria in cases of spontaneous and recurrent miscarriages and after exposure to
radiation, chemical mutagens, teratogenic noxes, and intra-
uterine infections. Relevant results from new research work
completed since the publication of the first edition have been
included. Apart from this, we have altered a few passages and
illustrations for the sake of clarity. We would like to express
our gratitude for the comments and criticisms of many of
our colleagues which have helped us in preparing this new
edition.

Preface to the
First Edition

"An ounce of prevention is worth a pound of cure."

In medicine the truth of this statement is so self-evident that it is simply taken for granted; and yet it has become mere lip-service for many a doctor, since his work is almost exclusively concerned with the treatment of those who are already ill. This applies not only to the treatment of patients but even more to that of entire families. Many doctors are as yet unaware that the appearance of serious, sometimes fatal diseases can be avoided by preventing the conception of sick human beings. Our knowledge of genetics permits the relatively accurate prediction, based on statistical probability, of the recurrence of genetic defects (anomalies) and diseases within families.

Our patients are frequently aware that such predictions are possible. In an effort to prevent the birth of defective children they try to inform themselves. However, in the practice of the individual doctor this sort of inquiry does not occur with such frequency that he is forced to concern himself systematically with these problems. Should he be confronted with such an inquiry, the doctor conscientiously tries to recall what he has read—once upon a time. In many cases the doctor's actual contact with genetics has occurred so long ago that he has forgotten most of the particulars, or genetics was never taught when he was at university. Consequently, the practicing physician usually has no exact knowledge on which to base his advice. Either he evades the problem with vague generalities, or he remembers various statements about "heredity" that almost always lead to false conclusions.

From discussions with our colleagues, we know that they recognize the problems and worry about them, but simply do not have the time to thoroughly study the highly specialized genetic literature available.

This book is an attempt to fill this void. We have made an effort to keep it as short and clear as possible and to limit it to the important and most frequent genetic abnormalities. In particular, we have tried to take into consideration the difficulties of the average student in understanding genetic logic and to eliminate the most common errors.

This guide is not designed to provide more than basic information. No reader will arise from the study of this volume as an expert genetic counselor. That requires, in this as in all other sciences, knowledge of the highly specialized literature as well as extensive experience. Some geneticists therefore take the position that the general practitioner (or specialist in any other field of medicine) cannot possibly give proper genetic counsel to his patients. Because he is not a genetics expert, he should, without exception, refer all such cases to the geneticist. This point of view would condemn this guide as potentially more harmful than helpful in that it might increase the cases of well-meaning error as well as encouraging those who are not competent in this field to deal with problems which are beyond their capacity.

We, obviously, do not share this pessimistic standpoint. In our opinion, there are cases in which an interested and informed general practitioner can give fully adequate counsel. In these cases it is of great advantage to the effectiveness of the advice that family doctor who has the confidence of his patient(s) also carry out the counseling. Opposed to these clear cases are the highly complex ones which exceed this guide's limitations. In such cases the doctor must recognize the limits of his knowledge and consult a genetic counseling clinic or a specialist. Exactly where the limits are to be found in a specific case must be left to the conscience of the individual doctor. We are confident that the doctor, once he has become aware that genetic problems are often very complex indeed, will preferably consult the specialist too often rather than too little. Even if the doctor has come to the conclusion that he cannot responsibly counsel any such case, the information in this guide will help him to understand the nature of the problem with which the specialist is confronted. It will, moreover, help him to recognize problems which require the specialist and allow him to aid the latter in gathering relevant information.

We sincerely hope that this guide will prove helpful to many practicing physicians and beneficial for patients and their families.

Contents

1 Appearances Deceive

In this first chapter we have illustrated many of the problems of analysis with a specific case history. This approach necessitated the use of various terms and concepts, the exact meanings of which are defined and explained in later chapters. Readers are advised not to despair but to reread the first chapter after they have carefully read the rest. We recommend Chapter 2 as the starting point and Chapter 1 as the conclusion for those readers who have had little or no previous contact with genetics.

Example 1: A 25-year-old university graduate requests counseling. He himself is mentally and physically normal, and his fiancé, a girl of good family, is equally normal, genetically speaking. The girl's parents, responsible people, were interested in their future son-in-law's family. To their horror, they discovered the situation illustrated in the pedigree in Fig. 1.1. Two half-sisters of the young

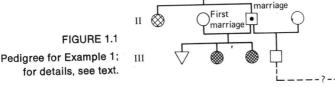

FIGURE 1.1

Pedigree for Example 1; for details, see text.

man suffer from Hurler's disease; they are both badly malformed. The father and grandfather of the proband both manifest Dupuytren's contracture of the hand, and added to all this, the father's sister suffers from a congenital dislocation of the hip.

It will surprise no one that the girl's father began to doubt the advisability of such a marriage. His decision to consult a specialist must be evaluated as a responsible attempt to base his opinion on fact rather than on prejudice. The two specialists consulted were doctors whose respective fields of specialization appeared to validate their opinion. One doctor advised against the marriage on the grounds that such a family history involved too great a risk for potential children. The other doctor stated that Hurler's disease belongs to the category of generalized dysostoses and that this type of disease is known to have genetic causes; therefore, the marriage is ill-advised.

This information resulted in massive parental pressure, on the girl's side, directed at breaking the engagement. The situation developed into a suicide attempt on the girl's part, which fortunately remained an attempt only. At this point, the young man turned to genetic family counseling as a last resort. A careful genetic analysis of the situation made it possible to reassure the young man that, genetically speaking, there were no serious objections to the marriage. The same conclusion could also be presented in good conscience to the parents of the girl. *The chance that children from this marriage will suffer from a serious genetic defect is only negligibly higher than that of children from the average population.*

This somewhat surprising conclusion requires a careful study of the pedigree shown in Fig. 1.1.

Hurler's Disease   The most serious defect involved is Hurler's disease. If the prospective children of a marriage were likely to suffer from this disease, this alone would make such a union inadvisable. Therefore, the first question to be answered is "How great is the risk that a child from this marriage will have Hurler's disease?" In order to answer this question, the mode of inheritance for the disease must be known. In this case, the mode is known to be autosomal-recessive. This means that, in order to manifest itself, a disease requires the patient to be homozygous for the defective allele in question. He must carry the defective gene on two homologous chromosomes. Of these two homologous chromosomes, one comes from his mother (II, 2), the other from his father (II, 3); see Fig. 1.1., and also Chapter 5. Both parents must therefore have the defective gene. Since neither parent personally manifests the disease, one may conclude that each possesses, at worst, only one defective gene; i.e., they are heterozygous. Consequently, every child resulting from such a union has a 25% chance of being homozygous for the defective gene, and therefore manifesting the disease; a 50% chance of being heterozygous and therefore personally unaffected; and a 25% chance of being homozygous for the normal allele.

Keeping this in mind, let us review the young man's particular situation. First of all, he himself is definitely not suffering from this disease and therefore cannot be homozygous for the defective gene. Added to this is the fact that he is merely the half-brother of the affected members of the family; he has a different mother. His father must be heterozygous, but his mother in all likelihood is not, for this genetic defect is very rare. Since the proband can only have received one of the two homologous chromosomes of his father, of which only one carries the defective gene, there is a 50% chance that he too carries the defective gene and is therefore heterozygous.

Let us now consider his fianceé. As far as we know, her family is entirely normal. She is in no way related to her future spouse. Children from this union would only be affected with Hurler's disease—and then with a 25% probability for each child—if the girl were heterozygous as well. Since there are no factors indicating that this is the case, the probability that it is so is no higher than the risk for every other human being in the average population.

This chance can be calculated, provided one possesses the frequency of the disease figures for the mean population. In this case, we have no exact data, but one thing is certain: this particular anomaly is very rare. (Should difficulties arise in understanding the calculations below, we suggest that the reader refer to the discussion of the Hardy-Weinberg Law and the concept of gene frequency in the population in Chapter 5.)

Estimating the population frequency of this anomaly at roughly 1 : 100,000, this means a gene frequency of $q = \sqrt{10^{-5}}$ = 0.00317 and a heterozygote frequency of $2\,pq = 0.00634$, or about 6:1000. At this point, we will calculate the probability that both parents are heterozygous. This is done as follows:

0.5 (for the young man) $\times$ 0.006 (for his fianceé) = 0.003 or about 3 : 1000 for both being heterozygous. Should the union actually be one of these three, then each child has a 25% chance of manifesting the anomaly. Thus the predictable risk is calculated as 0.002 $\times$ 0.25 = <1 : 1000 for future children.

As already stated, this calculation is a very rough estimate. More accurate figures would require precise knowledge of the gene frequency instead of mere approximations. Nonetheless, even this rough estimate demonstrates one point very clearly: the increase in the risk for children of this union is very small. It is certainly insufficient justification for a "no-marriage" counsel. This becomes even more valid when we consider that every unborn child runs a 1 to 2% risk of being born with some sort of congenital malformation or hereditary disease. Compared to this risk, inherent in the conception of any child, the increased danger for a child from this union is negligible.

Dupuytren's Contracture

However, Hurler's disease is not the only genetic anomaly in this family. Apart from this, the father and grandfather have manifested Dupuytren's contracture of the hands. Experience classifies Dupuytren's contracture as having an autosomal dominant mode of inheritance. In other words, the genetic defect already manifests itself in the heterozygous patient, and will be passed on to half his children (Chapter 3). However, the disease does not manifest itself to the same extent in every individual; the "expressivity" is variable. Furthermore, Dupuytren's contracture usually does not become apparent until middle age or later, and even then not always; penetrance is not complete. The disease also shows signs of a sex limitation in that more men than women are affected.

Given the above information, our evaluation of this young man's situation is as follows: so far the anomaly has not appeared, but the proband has not yet reached the "dangerous" age. Since his father and grandfather are both affected, there is a 50% chance that the son will develop the trait sooner or later. Should the anomaly manifest itself, it will prove that the proband is heterozygous for this gene, and that, on the average, 50% of his children will inherit it. His sons, if heterozygous, will then, at some time in later life, develop Dupuytren's contracture; his daughters, even if they do possess the gene, have a chance of not being affected, in spite of it.

In other words, as long as we cannot be sure that the proband himself is heterozygous, the calculated risk for his children is as follows: for his sons, $\frac{1}{2} \times \frac{1}{2} = \frac{1}{4}$; for his daughters, $\frac{1}{2} \times \frac{1}{2} \times m = \frac{1}{4} \times m$, m being the manifestation probability in relation to women; therefore, the absolute risk for daughters is less than 25%.

Nonetheless, a genetic risk of 25% is anything but negligible. Does not such a considerable danger indicate that the union is ill-advised, or at least that this couple should not have children? Were the genetic defect a really serious one, the answer to this question would undoubtedly be "yes." Dupuytren's contracture, however, is only a minor anomaly that does not seriously limit the affected individual. Moreover, it can be corrected surgically. The disease is not such that it affects either the patient's life expectancy or his capacity to live a full life.

This means, that, although it should be mentioned that children from this union are likely to develop this anomaly, on sound consideration, most people will not be deterred from having children.

Hip Dislocation   The remaining problem to be considered is the case of congenital dislocation of the hip in the proband's aunt. Her case, insofar as we have been able to discover, is the only one in the family. This is quite usual. Research with numerous series has demonstrated that the development of this anomaly does involve a genetic component, probably sometimes the one responsible for the comparatively shallow development of the articular cavity of the hip; but the genetic component is not the only determining factor for this defect, a discovery based on research with a series of twins. When an anomaly is exclusively determined by the genetic factor, identical twins (monozygotic twins, MT) as a rule display the exact same defects (are concordant). Monozygotic twins are, after all, derived from a single egg, fertilized by a single sperm, thus giving both an identical complement of genes.

Table 1.1 shows the collected data of the twin research series (random series) in relation to congenital dislocation of the hip. Monozygotic twins show a noticeably higher concordance than diszygotic twins, a fact that points to a genetic cause. However, the concordance is by no means absolute, which proves that the appearance of this defect involves other factors as well.

Apart from this evidence, congenital dislocation of the hip belongs to that group of defects for which no simple mode of inheritance has been established (other considerations indicate that this is likely to be a permanent state of affairs). For this reason, one cannot even derive the percentile risk involved in the various degrees of relationship through a theoretical segregation figure; all predictions must be based on empirical statistics.

There are records of random series indicating the frequency with which this anomaly appears within the various degrees of relationship. On the basis of these figures, it is possible to calculate the empiric or statistical risk. Table 1.2 gives a brief summary of the figures derived from such research (see also Table 9.1).

But to return to our specific case, the particular question that concerns us is the empiric risk that the patient's great-

Table 1.1   Frequency of Congenital Dislocation of the Hip in Mono- and Dizygotic Twins

	n	Number of concordant cases	%	Frequency of bilaterally affected cases
MT	29	12	41.4%	41%
DT	109	3	2.8	

Data from Idelberger (1951).

nephews and nieces will inherit the anomaly. As a quick glance at Table 1.2 shows, there are very few examples in the series referring to such a remote relationship. But even close relatives have only a small chance of manifesting the anomaly. Thus we conclude that the risk that a future child of this union will be born with a congenital dislocation of the hip is only negligibly, if at all, increased compared to the risk for the mean population. Thus, the possibility of this disease does not constitute a serious objection to the marriage either.

A brief summary of the pedigree analysis (Fig. 1.1) would be as follows: *The only real "danger" for future children consists of the potential appearance of Dupuytren's contracture at an advanced age. This risk in no way constitutes a reason to advise against the marriage.*

General Rules of Counseling The following general rules applying to genetic family counseling can be deduced from the preceding case history.

1. There are still only a very small number of people who seek genetic family counseling, but these few are, as a rule, particularly responsible people. Therefore, the decisions they arrive at as a result of our advice will likely be basic to their entire way of life. Frequently, it is their future life and happiness that hangs in the balance. Because the consequences are so far-reaching, *these people deserve advice based on the best and newest information that our research and knowledge in genetics has to offer.*

2. It is always wrong to conclude the existence of a "dangerous" genetic liability on the basis of the appearance of several anomalies in the same family. The most important general principle in genetic family counseling is that *there is no such thing as nonspecific "dangerous genetic liability." There are only specific diseases and specific modes of inheritance.* Every case requires a careful record of the proband's pedigree, in which all the members of the family, whether normal or otherwise, appear. The specific method for such a pedigree writeup will be discussed later.

Once the pedigree has been recorded, the facts should be analyzed and evaluated according to the specific knowledge

Table 1.2 Empiric Risk figures for Congenital Dislocation of the Hip

Number and sex of proband	Brother	Sister	Son	Daughter	Uncle	Aunt	Nephew	Niece	Cousin male	Cousin female
♂, 37	0/25 0%	2/29 6.89%	0/3 0%	0/7 0%	0/84 0%	0/91 0%	0/16 0%	1/13 7.59%	0/89 0%	0/94 0%
♀, 219	1/177 0.56%	11/176 6.25%	0/48 0%	5/45 11.11%	1/445 0.22%	0/81 0%	2/100 2%	0/601 0%	2/614 0.33%	

Data from Carter (1964); data combined from two series.

of medical genetics. Should the pedigree show several anomalies, the first step is to discover whether all the anomalies have a common genetic root, or whether it is sheer coincidence that they occur together. Of course, this question cannot be decided on the evidence given in the pedigree alone, no matter how accurate. The other prerequisite is a thorough knowledge of the genetic literature dealing with the subject including possible statistical evidence concerning particular combinations of anomalies within familes or in the same person. (This is particularly applicable when the modes of inheritance have not been established.) The pedigree discussed in Fig. 1.1 is an example of an accidental combination of anomalies. There is no evidence suggesting that the suspicious simultaneous occurrence in the same family of Hurler's disease, Dupuytren's contraction, and a congenital dislocation of the hip has a common genetic root.

A group of which the contrary would be true is the group of atopic diseases. Atopic dermatitis, bronchial asthma, and hay fever occur too frequently within the same families for this combination to be accidental. One can often observe all three in the same patient at the same or at different times.

But a surface similarity or even the same general classification in some nosological system does not constitute grounds for assuming a common mode of inheritance. For example, combined harelip and cleft palate on the one hand, and simple cleft palate on the other, are in most cases genetically independent.

3. Exact diagnosis is the basic prerequisite of any form of counseling. This self-evident statement is meant to emphasize the absolute necessity of *differentiating between a genetic disease and a phenotypically similar clinical condition.* Originally, Hurler's disease had been considered a disease entity. It is now recognized that the group of mucopolysaccharidoses comprises at least six different types. The name Hurler's disease has been retained for the autosomal-recessive type 1. Table 1.3 gives the essential features of the various types. Of particular importance is the discrimination of Hurler's disease from the sex-linked type 2 (Hunter's). Had the two patients in the pedigree in Fig. 1.1 been male instead of female, one would have been obliged to consider this possibility. The various symptoms do permit a differentiation between the two anomalies, but only with a relative degree of certainty. If, however, it had been concluded that the anomaly was Hunter's type, then the patients would have received the defective gene from the mother. Since the proband has a different mother, and he himself is definitely not affected, he could not then be even a carrier for this gene.

In human genetics, experience has consistently shown that a careful analysis of a clinical condition generally regarded as typical and straightforward usually leads to a reclassification into several—often many—genetically independent types. An

Table 1.3

Catalog no.	Designation	Clinical features	Genetics	Excessive urinary MPS	Enzyme deficient
25280	MPS I H — Hurler's syndrome	Early clouding of cornea, grave manifestations, death usually before age 10	Homozygous for MPS I H gene	Dermatan sulfate Heparan sulfate	α-L-iduronidase
	MPS I S — Scheie's syndrome	Stiff joints, cloudy cornea, aortic regurgitation, normal intelligence, ?normal life-span		Dermatan sulfate Heparan sulfate	α-L-iduronidase
	MPS I H/S — Hurler–Scheie compound	Phenotype intermediate between Hurler and Scheie	Genetic compound of MPS I H and I S genes	Dermatan sulfate Heparan sulfate	α-L-iduronidase
30990	MPS II A — Hunter's syndrome, severe	No clouding of cornea, milder course than in MPS IH, but death usually before age 15	Hemizygous for X-linked gene	Dermatan sulfate Heparan sulfate	Sulfo-iduronide sulfatase
	MPS II B — Hunter's syndrome, mild	Survival to 30's to 50's, fair intelligence	Hemizygous for X-linked allele for mild form	Dermatan sulfate Heparan sulfate	Sulfo-iduronide sulfatase
25290	MPS III A — Sanfilippo's syndrome A	Identical phenotype	Homozygous for Sanfilippo A gene	Heparan sulfate	Heparan sulfate sulfatase

				Homozygous for Sanfilippo B (at different locus)	Heparan sulfate	N-acetyl-α-D glucosaminidase
25292	MPS III B	Sanfilippo's syndrome B	Mild somatic, severe central nervous system effects	Homozygous for Sanfilippo B (at different locus)	Heparan sulfate	N-acetyl-α & -β glucosaminidase
25300	MPS IV	Morquio's syndrome (probably more than one allelic form)	Severe bone changes of distinctive type, cloudy cornea, aortic regurgitation	Homozygous for Morquio gene	Keratan sulfate	?Chondroitin sulfate sulfatase
25320	MPS V	Vacant (now MPS I S)				
	MPS VI A	Maroteaux–Lamy's syndrome, severe form	Severe osseous and corneal change, normal intellect	Homozygous for M–L gene	Dermatan sulfate	Arylsulfatase B
25322	MPS VI B	Maroteaux–Lamy's syndrome, mild form	Mild osseous and corneal change, normal intellect	Homozygous for allele at M–L locus	Dermatan sulfate	Arylsulfatase B
	MPS VII	β-glucuronidase deficiency (more than one allelic form?)	Hepatosplenomegaly, dysostosis multiplex, white cell inclusions, mental retardation	Homozygous for mutant gene at beta-glucuronidase locus	Dermatan sulfate	β-glucuronidase

Data from McKusick (1975).

analysis of the clinical picture taken together with the known modes of inheritance often makes this necessary.

In genetic diseases in which the exact biochemical defect at the root of all the symptoms can be established, this differentiating process goes even further. The fact is that phenotypically almost identical conditions may have totally different and independent genetic causes. We call it "genetic heterogeneity."

It is these similarities that make an accurate diagnosis so difficult—and so very important—if one wishes to avoid erroneous counsel.

4. There is one more aspect to counseling that arises from the appearance of Dupuytren's contraction in the example above. For the actual counseling, not only the degree but also the kind of risk involved is important. After all, the degree of disability involved is a considerable factor in such decisions. The smaller the potential defect, the greater the risk that prospective parents will be willing to take. Many geneticists believe, however, that all value judgments should be avoided in counseling, and that advising the parties concerned of the facts and the degree of risk involved is the total extent of their function. The final decision belongs to those involved, and personal opinions have no place in factual information. Granting that the final decision is up to the parties involved, we still feel that the counselor should not evade the responsibility of taking a personal stand. We will deal with the personal and psychological aspects of counseling later, but that these are important and play a considerable, if not decisive, role, no one will deny.

We would like to enumerate once more the question that must be asked every time that a confrontation with a specific genetic problem occurs, in the order in which they must be answered:

1. What is the exact diagnosis?
2. The pedigree: what are the known facts and the results of Medical examination?
3. The proband's relationship (or that of potential children) to the patient.
4. Has the mode of inheritance been established?
5. Are there research records giving the empiric risk figures?

The answer to these questions will provide the data for the *specific genetic prognosis.* In order to evaluate these facts correctly, the doctor must now ask himself:

6. How severe is the anomaly?

The remaining questions are the self-critical, searching questions common to all medical consultation.

7. Are further examinations of the proband or his relatives possible or indicated?

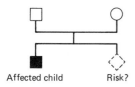

Affected child   Risk?

FIGURE 1.2

8. Am I capable, with my knowledge, of dealing responsibly with the matter by myself, or should I consult another specialist, particularly a geneticist?

The following chapters will, we hope, make the answer to these questions easier for the general practitioner confronted with this sort of problem. We are going to discuss the situations which, according to experience, arise most frequently, and attempt to illustrate the method of dealing with them through examples. But before we do this, we are simply going to give one example that will demonstrate the many considerations which arise and must be dealt with from case to case. This example is, at the same time, the most common of all situations: a child with a defect is born into a normal family.

The parents want to know with what degree of probability the next child is likely to be affected as well. The most important possibilities are enumerated in the following tabulation:

The mode of inheritance for the defect in question	The probability of further affected children
1. An autosomal-recessive genetic defect (see Chapter 5)	25%
2. An autosomal-dominant genetic defect with a high degree of penetrance ("new mutation," see Chapter 4)	$\approx$ 0%
3. A rare, sex-linked recessive genetic defect; the patient is male (see Chapter 6)	Sisters $\approx$ 0% Brothers $\leqq$ 50%
4. Chromosome anomaly (see Chapter 7)	From less than 1% up to (in rare cases) 100%.
5. A genetic anomaly not based on any simple mode of inheritance (see Chapters 8 and 10)	In accordance with empirical risk figures; often less than 10%.
6. A nongenetic malformation, given normal circumstances, i.e., no clinical illness or serious disturbance in the reproductive system of the mother pointing to a constant jeopardy for future children.	Generally no higher than the risk for the average population.

2 Recording a Family Medical History or Pedigree

A careful and detailed health history of the family is the basic prerequisite for any form of genetic counseling. It is essential to have detailed information about the proband's relatives even when the proband himself is clearly suffering from a genetic defect of which the mode of inheritance has, ostensibly, been established. In genetics, there is always the possibility that a particular family will prove to be an exception. It happens, for instance, that a genetic defect, generally considered as autosomal-recessive, will be passed on as a dominant trait in some families. This, of course, also demonstrates that the same clinical disease has a separate genetic cause. A detailed pedigree gives us the necessary basic information for all further genetic considerations. It simplifies matters for oneself and the potentially required geneticist if the pedigree is drawn up with the symbols in common usage, such as those given in Figs. 2.1a, b.

The rules to be observed in recording a pedigree are few and simple, but they are essential. As a matter of principle, the record must show all the children of a sibship, whether defective or normal. Wherever accurate information is lacking —i.e., the person asked cannot definitely state the number of children or their sex—this too should be noted. A pedigree is supposed to show the various births in their proper order. If this can no longer be ascertained, the ambiguous quality of the information should be recorded as shown in Fig. 2.2

If, for some reason, the recorded order differs from the actual and known order, then this must be pointed out as well. It is also very important to try to locate stillbirths and miscarriages in a sibship as correctly as possible. Although infor-

(a)

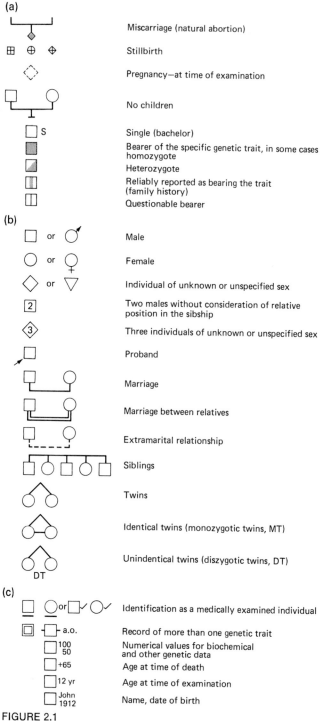

Miscarriage (natural abortion)

Stillbirth

Pregnancy—at time of examination

No children

S — Single (bachelor)

Bearer of the specific genetic trait, in some cases homozygote

Heterozygote

Reliably reported as bearing the trait (family history)

Questionable bearer

(b)

☐ or ♂ — Male

○ or ♀ — Female

◇ or ▽ — Individual of unknown or unspecified sex

2 — Two males without consideration of relative position in the sibship

⟨3⟩ — Three individuals of unknown or unspecified sex

Proband

Marriage

Marriage between relatives

Extramarital relationship

Siblings

Twins

Identical twins (monozygotic twins, MT)

Unindentical twins (diszygotic twins, DT)

DT

(c)

☐ ○ or ☐✓ ○✓ — Identification as a medically examined individual

☐ ☐- a.o. — Record of more than one genetic trait

☐ 100 50 — Numerical values for biochemical and other genetic data

☐ +65 — Age at time of death

☐ 12 yr — Age at time of examination

☐ John 1912 — Name, date of birth

FIGURE 2.1

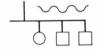

FIGURE 2.2

mation on these points is frequently particularly vague, it could become a central factor in a later evaluation.

For the sake of clarity, it is desirable, as a rule, to arrange the pedigree with the paternal line on the left-hand side and the maternal line on the right. Therefore, it may simplify matters in the diagram to place the father in question at the end of his sibship, outside his proper place in the birth order. The same reasoning applies for placing the mother at the beginning of hers. Nonetheless, the actual place should be marked as well. It is also helpful, for the sake of later discussions, if the name and date of birth of the person appear on either side of the symbol referring to him.

In numbering the pedigree, it is common practice to indicate successive generations with Roman numerals (descending order), and to indicate the order within the generation with Arabic numerals (left to right). Other numbering systems are acceptable, provided they are used consistently so that the clarity of the diagram does not suffer. It is important that every member of the family be clearly identified. Figure 3.2 gives an example.

Conflicting reports of past happenings are standard during the first information-gathering sessions. This means that the actual numbering is only possible in the final draft of the pedigree. For this reason, it is particularly important to keep a separate list containing the most important data.

1. The number within the pedigree.
2. Family name, first name, and, if applicable, maiden name.
3. Date and place of birth (date of death).
4. Address.
5. Name of the proband's doctor and hospital and their addresses.
6. A brief medical case history of the proband.
7. The specific nature of the inquiry and, if applicable, the relevant data concerning the specific genetic problem in the family.
8. Family members known to be unaffected.

Such a detailed record of a family pedigree requires time and patience, but it is absolutely essential. It cannot be sufficiently emphasized that no amount of care in the later evaluation will balance carelessness at this stage.

In order to maintain a strict standard of accuracy, it is generally advisable to take down all the particulars for each family member separately. Once this has been done, the information should be verified and expanded or qualified by questioning other members of the family. The sources of the information are best recorded as well. Generally speaking, when it comes to information concerning past generations or distant relatives, grandmothers tend to be a gold mine. Naturally, inquiries are best directed at both marriage partners, just as the resultant counsel will later be discussed—preferably written down as well—in the presence of both.

Insofar as it is at all possible, individuals whose specific condition is important to the outcome of the genetic evaluation should be medically examined. If that proves impossible, their own doctors should be questioned for the relevant data. From time to time, an additional examination by a specialist will be required, but one should never forget that in the case of some illnesses a carefully recorded medical history is more accurate and valuable than the results of any single medical examination or test. If we take epilepsy as an example, the results of an examination might be perfectly normal if it took place in the interval between attacks. In many cases, however, an examination is of paramount importance and it is essential to pay attention to even the most minute deviation from the normal. In some cases of incomplete penetrance, very minor or even microsymptoms will be the only evidence identifying the individual as a gene carrier.

In general, it can be assumed that a person actually seeking genetic counsel is prepared to supply accurate information to the best of his knowledge and ability. Unfortunately, the same is not necessarily true of his relatives, and it does happen that the proband himself is unable or unwilling to be unreservedly open. For instance, an accepted family interpretation of an anomaly as due to an accident can make it very difficult to trace the actual roots of the particular incident.

The question remains: How far back is one required to go? There is simply no single answer to this question. Ultimately, the extent of the research will be decided by the requirements of the particular case. It depends upon (a) the kind of genetic defect that confronts us, (b) which mode of inheritance applies, and (c) how definitely the mode of inheritance has been ascertained. Again, the basic requirements remain the same. With few exceptions, an analysis must include the detailed record of the proband's siblings and parents, the parents' siblings and their children, as well as the proband's nephews and nieces, should they exist. The same information about the (prospective) spouse's corresponding set of relatives must be obtained and considered. If circumstances so dictate, the grandparents must be included in the pedigree. Above all, the question of possible consanguinity must be raised and answered in relation to each set of parents. As far as practical counseling is concerned, it is very important to ascertain whether there exists any blood relationship between the families of the engaged (married) couple. Consanguinity also arises as a problem if both partners originate from the same village or small town.

Frequently, it will not be possible to obtain, much less verify, all the necessary data. More often than not, one is obliged to base one's final counsel on the restricted information supplied by the proband and, possibly, his partner. Under these circumstances, all counsel is of course provisional. It must be strongly emphasized that in such a situation, the validity of the evaluation depends entirely upon the accuracy of the information received and the truth of plausible assumptions about other family members that one may have had to make.

3 The Autosomal Dominant Mode of Inheritance

The Mendelian laws of heredity apply to human beings as to all other living creatures. The genes are present on every single chromosome of the 46 that each human being possesses in every single cell of his body. Two of these chromosomes are sex chromosomes (sex-determining; see Chapter 7, Fig. 7.2) and the remaining 44 are known as autosomes. Traits determined by genetic information on these chromosomes are called autosomally inherited. The autosomes pair according to their shape and the members contain the same gene loci (homologous chromosomes). Consequently, every autosomal gene locus occurs twice in every cell of the body. If both loci possess the same genetic information, the individual is homozygous (ομος = identical). But if the two gene loci carry different information (alleles), the individual may have one normal gene locus paired with a corresponding gene that carries a different allele. The individual will then be heterozygous (ετερός = different). In the case of a simple mode of inheritance, the individual may therefore be homozygous for the normal gene, homozygous for the defective gene, or he may possess each gene in a single dose and therefore be heterozygous for this gene locus.

In the formation of germ cells, the autosomes are so distributed that every germ cell contains one chromosome of each pair and consequently possesses a single edition of the genetic information for each gene locus. Apart from special cases (i.e., linkage), which are of secondary importance in this discussion, the distribution of genes (alleles) to the gametes seems to be arbitrary and according to the laws of probability. Even in the mating process, the laws of chance finally decide which one of millions of sperm will fertilize the ovum. It is a matter of total indifference after this which partner contrib-uted which chromosome or allele; in other words, whether a gene originally came in the ovum or the sperm. For this rea-son, possible gene combinations and the probability of their occurrence can best be tabulated in the checkerboard formula of "free" or "chance" combinations (Fig. 3.1).

Experimental genetics strictly defines the dominant mode of inheritance as the situation in which a single dose of a gene is quite sufficient to allow the trait thus governed full expres-sion. The heterozygote for such a gene will be phenotypically identical with the homozygote. It is impossible to differentiate between them in terms of physical differences.

This rather strict definition has been dropped in human genetics for purely practical reasons. For one thing, with rare genetic defects, homozygous cases are virtually unknown and the exact correspondence between the two genotypes is thus unverifiable. For another, whenever it is possible to definitely distinguish the two genotypes, the homozygote for a defec-tive gene is often noticeably more affected than his hetero-zygote counterpart. In order to stay within the limits of the

FIGURE 3.1. Combination probability calculation for the autosomal-dominant mode of inheritance.

Genotypes of parents:

AA	Gametes	
AA	A	A
A	AA	AA
A	AA	AA

Genotypes of children: AA, AA, AA, AA

Expected result: AA
              analog: a a

Genotypes of parents:

aa	Gametes	
Aa	a	a
a	aa	aa
A	Aa	Aa

Genotypes of children: aa, Aa, aa, Aa

Expected result: 2 X aa + 2 X Aa
                 1 : 1

Genotypes of parents:

Aa	Gametes	
Aa	A	a
A	AA	Aa
a	Aa	aa

Genotypes of children: AA, Aa, Aa, aa

Expected result: AA + 2 X Aa + aa
               1 : 2 : 1

Genotypes of parents:

aa	Gametes	
aa	A	A
a	Aa	Aa
a	Aa	Aa

Genotypes of children: Aa, Aa, Aa, Aa

Expected result: Aa

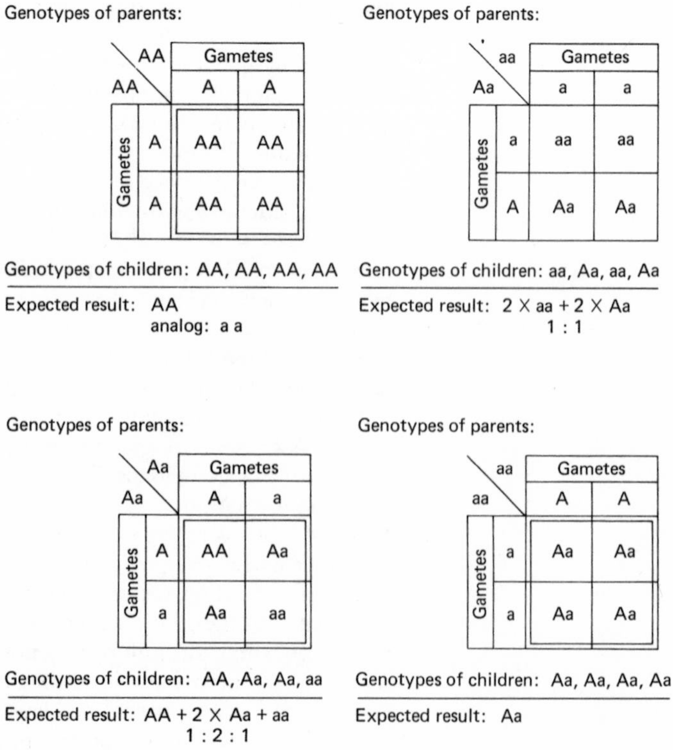

definition, one would be obliged to postulate an "intermediary" mode of inheritance, and absolute distinctions would still be impossible.

It has therefore become common usage to define a disease or defect as having a dominant mode of inheritance when the heterozygotes show a distinct variation from the norm. It should be pointed out that the categories of the autosomal-dominant or autosomal-recessive mode of inheritance represent abstractions dictated by practical necessity. They only approximate an accurate picture of the biological facts.

The characteristics of the autosomal-dominant mode of inheritance (in human genetic terms) are these: (a) The trait is passed on via one of the parents to approximately $1/2$ their children. This means a 50% inheritance probability for every child of a trait bearer. (b) The inheritance is totally independent of the sex of the bearer or the heir. Both sexes are equally affected and the defective gene can have come from either father or mother.

Siblings or children of affected individuals who themselves show no sign of the trait and who have passed the age by which time the disease or defect usually manifests itself can assume that they are free of the defective gene. Consequently, their children are not endangered beyond the norm.

But, as always, there are qualifications. The statements above flatly presuppose that the trait in question will always make its appearance within a set time limit. Unfortunately, it frequently happens with diseases of the autosomal-dominant variety that an individual will inherit the defective gene and pass it on, while he himself remains phenotypically unaffected. For unknown reasons, the defect does not manifest itself, and we are confronted with a case of *incomplete penetrance*. Thus, the analysis of a particular case must always include consideration of the question of whether the specific defect has a history of complete penetrance or not. This information can be obtained through experience and from the figures in relevant genetic literature. Equally important, or even more so, is the pedigree of the family in question, provided that it can be traced back for a sufficient number of generations with sufficient certainty. Before a diagnosis of incomplete penetrance can be made, a thorough and exact medical examination of apparently unaffected family members is usually necessary.

There is yet another qualification. Let us look at the theory that the defect will manifest itself equally, irrespective of sex. It can and does happen that physiological or other reasons will make a disease far more dangerous for one sex than for the other, with the net result of a distinct severity variation between the sexes. It also happens that an inherited defect will make it impossible for a woman to complete a pregnancy. Thus, at least part of the manifestation is sex-limited.

Example 2 (see Fig. 3.2): Mother and son manifest almost identical bilateral hypoplasias of all five digits with more strongly affected ulnar rays. Numerous interphalangeal joints had stiffened and the flexibility of the wrists had been drastically reduced. The third to the fifth toes of both individuals were also hypoplastic. The X ray showed osseal fusion in the area of the aplastic interphalangeal joints as well as in the wrist and tarsal bones and that the short bones of the fingers and toes had shortened and thickened. An old photograph of the grandfather showed that he suffered from the same malformation of the hands, and three of his six children, according to reliable report, were similarly affected.

Despite the fact that the woman as well as her father had managed to find a way of living reasonably well with their disability, the woman decided against further children. If the question had been asked in time, the 50% probability for the son could have been predicted.

The classic case of an autosomal-dominant hereditary disease with full penetrance is easily recognizable as such, even by the layman. In such circumstances, very little family data will suffice for making a genetically sound prediction.

We know approximately 1200 traits, including the "normal" ones, with an autosomal-dominant mode of inheritance. A list of these traits can be found in McKusick's compendium (4th Ed., 1975), which appears regularly in new editions. With the dominant mode of inheritance, heterozygotes are also affected and are therefore easily recognized. Genetic counseling is at its most accurate and effective in these cases, and can prevent—provided that it occurs in time—the conception of further sick children. For this reason, those who wish to justify the introduction of general eugenic measures usually support their arguments with examples from this group of anomalies. The objection to this line of argument from the point of view of population genetics (i.e., the science of the distribution and the equilibrium of gene frequency in the general population) is that these severe autosomal-dominant defects, which manifest themselves at an early age, in particular frequently prevent the patient from propagation.

FIGURE 3.2. Pedigree for Example 2.

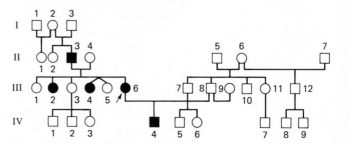

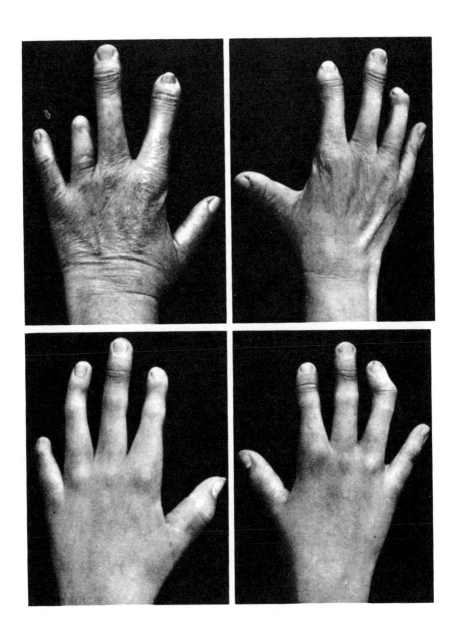

(a)

(b)

FIGURE 3.3. (a) Hands of the mother, proband III, 6; (b) hands of the son, proband IV, 4.

After Fuhrmann *et al.* (1965)

On the other hand, if the disease does not manifest itself until the normal procreative period has already passed, this general rule does not apply, and "natural selection" has no real effect. Under such conditions, the defective gene can multiply rapidly. An example of this is the history of Huntington's chorea, a progressive degeneration of the brain.

This gene, as far as we can tell, was brought into the United States by only three British immigrant families. Today, there are about 7000 affected individuals in the United States. The increase is frightening. This example, however, also serves to demonstrate that knowledge of the nature and causes of such a condition does lead people to limit their propagation without requiring legal coercion.

The real difficulty for genetic counseling in a case of Huntington's chorea lies in the fact that there are no overt symptoms, either at the marriageable age or throughout the normal procreative period, which indicate whether an offspring of a choreatic is heterozygous or not. There are as yet no test methods of any kind that would permit us to identify a heterozygote before the disease manifests itself—and the manifestation age for this disease is 40 or even later. Throughout the marriageable period, we can only estimate a 50% probability that a choreatic's son or daughter possesses the defective gene. Each of their children, even if they marry an unrelated partner from a normal family, would, with the same 50% probability, inherit the defective gene should his endangered parent actually prove heterozygous. With a history of complete penetrance for the disease, there is, while the genotype of the potentially affected parent remains unknown, a probability of $1/2 \times 1/2 = 1/4$ for each child.

Example 3 (see Fig. 3.4): When the diagnosis of Huntington's chorea had been established in the proband, the husband and the sons sought genetic counsel. The eldest son was just planning to get married. Further inquiry revealed that both the mother and an older sister of the proband suffered from a diagnosed chorea and that initial symptoms were beginning to manifest themselves in her brother. Since Huntington's chorea is transmitted as an autosomal dominant, the risk for every son of the proband is 50%. Provided

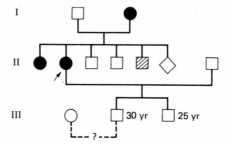

FIGURE 3.4
Pedigree for Example 3.

that his bride is not a relative, the risk for each of his prospective children is 0.5 × 0.5 = 25%. Prediction may become more precise in the future if a preclinical diagnosis of chorea should become possible.

With increasing knowledge of the genetic causes of the disease, and with the spread of family planning, the members of the affected families have, apparently, voluntarily limited the number of their chidren in comparison to the mean population. According to research done by Reed and Neel, this voluntary reduction holds true for those members who remained normal as well as for those in whom the disease manifested itself at a later date. As a consequence of this, the frequency of this gene must lessen. Fear of the disease (the children watching the affected parent getting progressively worse) plus sensible counseling has had a noticeable eugenic effect, although the individuals involved may very well have had only the welfare of their own families in mind.

For genetic family counseling, the degree of severity, or of limitation, imposed by any genetic disease is the decisive factor. We already referred to this in relation to the autosomal-dominant Dupuytren's contraction in Example 1, Chapter 1. In that case, the relatively minor disability caused by the disease plus the possibility of surgical correction made it possible to minimize and practically disregard the 25% risk evaluation. In the case of Huntington's chorea, there are no mitigating factors. The effects of the disease are devastating and, as yet, incurable.

In the case of autosomal-dominant diseases, actual counseling is usually made easier by the fact that the proband tends to be intimately acquainted with the disease. It has occurred within his own immediate family; he himself may be heterozygous. He is therefore usually quite capable of judging the severity of the effects and has definite opinions on whether he can answer for passing such a disease on to his children. Moreover, since the same inherited mutant is responsible for a given defect within the same kinship, the disease tends to follow a similar manifestation pattern in regard to its severity and its age of onset.

The basic rules for the autosomal-dominant mode of inheritance are as follows:

1. For every potential child of a patient with an autosomal-dominant hereditary disease manifesting complete penetrance, there is a 50% risk. Family members not suffering from the defect cannot pass it on; they are homozygous for the normal allele.

2. Children resulting from the union of two heterozygotes run a 75% risk of inheriting the anomaly. This figure includes the 25% risk that such a child will be homozygous for the

defective gene. Should the proband be the child of heterozygous parents, he himself might be homozygous. Should
this be the case, *all* his children will be heterozygous for the
gene in question.

These two simple general rules give the basic frame of
reference from which all further variations can be deduced.
Real difficulties arise only when there is an autosomal-dominant mode of inheritance with incomplete penetrance, or if
the individuals whose conditions are central to the analysis
have not yet passed the manifestation age. Even the phenotypically normal members of such a family have a calculable
chance of being heterozygous for the defective gene and can
thus become "donors" or carriers even if they never manifest
the disease themselves.

4 New Mutations and Phenocopies

The rules stated at the conclusion of the preceding chapter apply only when the specific disease in the family seeking advice is demonstrably subject to the autosomal-dominant mode of inheritance. Frequently, however, the symptoms of the proband will be identical to those observed in other families with the same anomaly in which the autosomal-dominant mode has been definitely established. Yet even the most painstaking research has failed to discover any further cases in the proband's family; of particular importance is the fact that there is nothing wrong with either of his parents. In situations of this kind, one of four explanations usually applies:

1. There is a phenotypically similar or identical disease that is subject to the autosomal-recessive mode of inheritance. Because we have apparently identical diseases with different modes of inheritance, we speak of "genetic heterogeneity," and this phenomenon is all too frequent. Whether this explanation is the correct one must be decided individually from case to case with the aid of knowledge derived from specialized genetic research publications. Should study of the relevant literature show that the problem is as yet unresolved because of insufficient research data, another factor that would point to the autosomal-recessive mode would be some degree of consanguinity between the parents, e.g., they are cousins. But, again, should the parents be unrelated, this does *not* exclude the possibility of an autosomal-recessive form of the anomaly. Fortunately, since there is no simple way of distinguishing the forms otherwise, there is a great deal of research literature dealing with the more common

defects that are subject to both modes and establishing the factors which differentiate the autosomal-recessive forms from the autosomal-dominants.

2. The second possibility is that of incomplete penetrance (see Chapter 3). In such a case, the trait, even if the parents seem unaffected, will be in evidence among the closer relatives such as siblings, grandparents, etc.

Besides these two possibilities, there are another two we will now discuss in detail: new mutations and phenocopies.

New Mutations   A gene may have mutated in the germ cell of either one of the parents, and should this germ cell be fertilized, the mutant will combine with its counterpart in other germ cell, thus forming a zygote. In consequence the zygote, and the human being developing from it, will be heterozygous for the mutation in question. The resulting trait or defect will manifest itself in the child and in its descendants should the mutation be autosomal-dominant. Figure 4.1 gives an example of such a pedigree; aniridia, as a rule, follows the autosomal-dominant mode of inheritance. As far as we know, neither phenocopies (see below) nor a phenotypically similar recessive form exists. Moreover, the evidence speaks conclusively for the autosomal-dominant mode of inheritance in this case. One only has to look at the children (Generation III) of the first affected individual in this family (Figure 4.1). As a rule, genetic family counseling becomes desirable as soon as a defective child is born into a hitherto normal family—in this case, a single sick child in Generation II. The birth of the other sick children in Generation III could have been predicted, and the original patient could have been warned of the risk involved in propagating himself. On the other hand, any anxiety on the part of the parents of generation I concerning the danger of

FIGURE 4.1. The first appearance of an autosomal-dominant trait (aniridia; bilaterally missing irises) caused by a new mutation in one of the germ cells of one of the parents. The original trait bearer in generation II passes the defective gene on to seven of his eleven children.

After Mollenbach (1947; cited by Vogel, 1961)

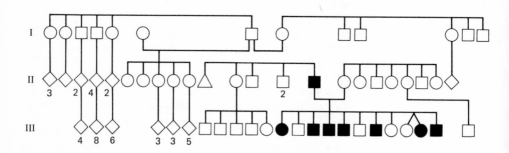

producing more defective children could have been allayed. A new mutation is an isolated occurrence, affecting only a single germ cell.

There is simply no evidence to support the theory of an increased probability of mutations in the other germ cells of the same person or his partner. The mutation probability (mutation rate) for the dominant gene or genes governing aniridia is, according to concurring estimates from Denmark and the U.S.A., about 2 to 3 in a million fertilized gametes.

With autosomal-dominant conditions, the ratio of new mutations to the sum total of cases differs from disease to disease. On the whole, the following common-sense rule applies: *The frequency ratio of new mutations to cases of established inheritance is directly proportional to the severity with which the resulting anomaly affects the patient's health at an early age and thus prevents him from propagating.*

The reasoning for this assertion is simple: if the individuals possessing a defective gene have fewer children than the population average, and if there are no new mutations, then the frequency of defective genes will consistently decrease from generation to generation until the defect dies out altogether. Since the serious dominant genetic defects have not died out, despite the fact that their existence demonstrably does and has reduced propagation on the part of the affected individuals, it is plausible to assume that new mutations occur to swell the thinning ranks. As the example showed, new mutations can actually be traced.

With the passing generations, an equilibrium of the gene frequency in the population establishes itself. This equilibrium implies that the number of genes eliminated by natural selection equals the number of new mutations for that specific gene. The fewer the children of last generation's trait bearers, the more trait bearers of the next generation will be new mutations, up to the extreme cases where the trait bearers never propagate themselves and therefore all new cases are new mutations. With this latter type, the distinction between new mutations and exogenously caused anomalies becomes impossible.

As an example, let us take retinoblastoma, a malignant eye tumor affecting little children. Until the practice of enucleation of the bulbus oculi was introduced by A. von Graefe a hundred years ago, all the patients simply died. It was not until there were survivors of the operation who had children that it became evident that some of the original cases were dominant new mutations. Examples of new mutations where the affected individuals, as a rule, simply do not reproduce and where the genetic cause is only established through rare exceptions to this rule are acrocephalosyndactyly (Apert's syndrome) and myositis ossificans. A contrary example of a severe dominant genetic disease where new mutations have never been established as such, with a reasonable degree of certainty, is Huntington's chorea. This disease is a pathological degeneration of the brain, especially of the extrapyramidal nuclei (Nucleus caudatus; putamen); the symptoms are spontaneous uncontrollable motion plus a marked deterioration of the patient's intellectual and psychological condition.

With this disease, the average manifestation age is somewhere in the fifth decade of the patient's life span, with considerable margin in both directions. Because of this, the patients have ample opportunity to propagate before the disease becomes manifest. That the chorea should be comparatively so widespread is astonishing nonetheless. Perhaps circumstances in the past made it possible for some of the affected individuals to produce more than the average number of children before the disease made its appearance.

The above-mentioned diseases are the extreme cases. Most of the hereditary anomalies with the autosomal-dominant mode of inheritance range somewhere between these in their estimated ratio of new mutations to hereditary cases. An example of such diseases is achondroplasia (dwarfism caused by a decrease in the growth of the epiphyses. The patients have a normal trunk but severely shortened extremities); another is Marfan's syndrome (dislocation of the crystalline lens; arachnodactyly; anomalies of the aorta and the heart); a third example is osteogenesis imperfecta, Lobstein's type (abnormal brittleness of the bones due to a defective bone formation combined with blue sclerae and, often, with inner-ear deafness as well). Another disease that belongs in this category is neurofibromatosis. In an extreme case, the patient's body can be covered with benign tumors (neurofibromata), whereas minor cases have only a few tumors but many café-au-lait colored spots. As a final example, we will mention dystrophia myotonica. This disease manifests itself through a tonus disturbance of the muscles (myotonia) together with progressive atrophy and other symptoms. For achondroplasia and for Apert's syndrome there seem to be a rare autosomal-recessive form. Such exceptions must be reckoned with in analyzing a particular case.

Example 4: At birth, the girl already gave evidence of a malformation syndrome. She had a tower head and syndactyly of all fingers and toes. Acrocephalosyndactyly (Apert's syndrome) was diagnosed and a chromosome examination followed. The examination, however, showed a normal karyotype. This result was disappointing but not surprising. Apert's syndrome is caused by a dominant new mutation and one does not expect structural anomalies. The chromosome examination, in fact, was carried out in the remote hope of discovering a chromosome deletion, thus gaining some idea as to the localization of the gene in question. Patients suffering from Apert's syndrome are usually so defective that procreation does not occur. This particular child died three days after birth.

A pedigree was taken (Fig. 4.2). The father was 29, the mother

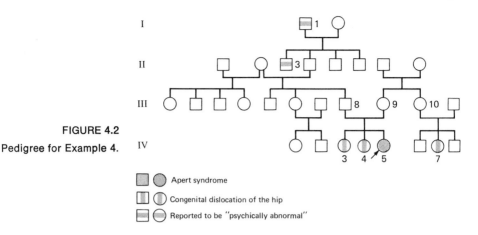

FIGURE 4.2
Pedigree for Example 4.

Apert syndrome
Congenital dislocation of the hip
Reported to be "psychically abnormal"

25, at the time of this birth. There were already two sisters, one 5, the other 4. The eldest had been born with a bilateral congenital dislocation of the hip which had been surgically corrected. The second child was put into a Fredjka splint at birth since she too gave evidence of a dislocated hip. Both girls now walk normally. A sister of the mother (III, 10) had three children, one of whom (IV, 7) also suffered from a congenital dislocation of the hip.

Further, apparently significant, information disclosed that the grandfather and an uncle of the father were "peculiar." They were, supposedly, "neurotic." A more particular inquiry showed that neither man had ever had either neurological or psychiatric treatment. Just the same, the relatives insisted that both were "neurotic." The grandfather had made life very difficult for his family, and the uncle, despite his college education, had never really amounted to much. His last job had been that of a tourist guide. At the moment (aged ca. 60) he was already living in an old people's home where he suffered from occasional fainting fits.

This kind of information is typical of the manner in which the average layman thinks of heredity. Of course, the possibility exists that the above information does contain a grain of truth in that the grandfather and the uncle were actually suffering from some unknown neurosis or psychological disturbance, but chances are that their "neurosis" was merely a case of personal oddities and weaknesses—not a rare occurrence among human beings. The information contained in these "facts" is totally irrelevant to genetic family counseling, except, of course, in cases where the proband is suffering from a hereditary mental illness.

There remains the one case of Apert's syndrome plus the three of congenital dislocation of the hip. As far as medical genetics is aware, these two diseases are not interrelated. Apart from this, according to the basic rule, genetic counseling must consider the two anomalies separately. The first question is as follows: What is the probability for another child with Apert's syndrome from this marriage?

Since, according to genetic knowledge, this case is one of a dominant new mutation and since we do not know of any factors that would constitute a "disposition" in one of the parents to produce mutations, we can assume that the probability concurs with the estimated risk figure for spontaneous mutations in the average population. In the case of Apert's syndrome, the mutation rate is estimated at 3 to 4 per million fertilized gametes. This chance is negligible, indeed, considering that every child runs an average risk of 1 to 2% of being born with a serious anomaly or malfunction.

Had the child itself matured and then asked the risk figures for its own children, the answer would have been quite different. Under these circumstances, the probability figures (this being a dominant mutation) stand at 50%.

The other problem in this family concerns the two children suffering from congenital dislocation of the hip. Empiric risk figures can be found in Table 1.2. According to this table, later children in families where one child is already suffering from this defect run an approximately 5% risk. In this family, however, there are already two cases, and the aunt has an affected child as well. We do not possess statistics for such a particularized situation, but common sense dictates that the risk will be about 10%. On the other hand, this particular defect does respond to early treatment, and this fact, too, should be pointed out.

Phenocopies   Even when a sporadic case shows all the symptoms of a dominant new mutation, it does not necessarily follow that this is the case. The further possibility exists that it is a phenocopy. This term was first coined by Richard Goldschmidt (1935), and it is defined as "an environmentally produced alteration in the manifestation of a genotype which copies the pattern of manifestation of another genotype" (Hadorn, 1961). Goldschmidt succeeded in producing numerous phenotypical deviations in drosophila by applying heat shocks to the wild type during various stages of their development. His "manufactured deviations" were very similar to the result of mutations.

It is possible to cause serious malformations during the very early stages of embryonic development in mammals as well. Observation indicates that this is also the case with human beings. But no experiments have ever produced anything remotely like the above-mentioned syndromes, which could be described as systemic malformations· When these occur in human beings, it can generally be assumed that the sporadic case is the result of a new mutation.

The problem changes when the defect in question is one such as a split hand or foot. In this area, there exist whole kinships with a regular dominant mode of inheritance and many affected members. Here, the split phenomenon tends to be equally expressed in all four extremities. A sporadic case with a similarly regular expressivity would be regarded as a dominant new mutation. Should, however, the split affect only one hand or foot—which is often the case—one would tend to suppose an exogenous cause. A rule of thumb is as follows: If malformations of the extremities (or other parts of the body) are bilateral and symmetrical, then a genetic cause is most likely. Should the malformation be unilateral and asymmetrical, chances are that there is an exogenous cause.

That this rule of thumb is at best an approximation and has many exceptions is shown by, for instance, the thalidomide embryopathy. Thalidomide is classed as a totally exogenous factor, and yet the malformations were often symmetrical. Apart from this, there is also the matter of incomplete penetrance. A genetic malformation, such as the split hand, with an autosomal-dominant mode of inheritance may manifest itself unilaterally.

One example, where it was possible to undertake a statistical analysis in an attempt to divide the new mutation from the phenocopies, is retinoblastoma. The results of this analysis and their general application to family counseling will be explained in greater detail at this point. The example demonstrates very clearly how carefully the particular circumstances of each case must be considered and differentiated even if the disease is the same.

To quickly summarize the general facts, retinoblastoma mostly affects children in infancy. Some 25% of them are bilaterally affected, either simultaneously or successively. The remaining 75% develop retinoblastoma unilaterally only. Without treatment, the tumor is practically 100% fatal. A spontaneous cure through necrosis of the tumor tissue is a very rare miracle indeed. The frequency figure for retinoblastoma is estimated at slightly less than 1 in 20,000 births.

Since it became possible to save the patients, an increase in the number of families with several affected members has been observed. A genetic analysis finally established an autosomal-dominant mode of inheritance with approximately 80% penetrance (see Chapter 3), i.e., among the heterozygotes about 20% remained unaffected for as yet inexplicable reasons. Oddly enough, however, only a very small minority (about 4%; figures vary somewhat) of affected individuals come from families where there are *any* other cases. The remaining 96% are apparently sporadic cases—and that is where the real genetic problem lies.

Is every case a dominant new mutation? If this were so, the chances for potential descendants would be rather grim; on the average, 50% would inherit the defective gene and of

these 50%, 80% would be affected—enough reason, in anyone's outlook, to advise against propagation.

A systematic series of examinations of children who were
operated at a sufficiently early age showed, fortunately, that
the situation is not quite as bad as that. All *bilaterally* affected
sporadic cases must, in fact, be regarded as new mutations,
and are subject to the above-mentioned conclusions. But
among the unilateral sporadic cases, only 15 to 20% are new
mutations. The remainder are unexplained phenocopies.

This reduces the risk for the children of unilateral sporadic
cases to 6 to 8% (= 40% of 15 to 20%). Again, we are as yet
unable to differentiate the dominant new mutations from the
nonhereditary phenocopies among these sporadic unilateral
cases.

The following rules for genetic family counseling can be
deduced from the preceding facts (see also Figs. 4.3 to 4.7).

1. In families where there are several cases of retinoblastoma, the terms of the problem are relatively simple: (a) The
inquirer himself has suffered from retinoblastoma (uni- or
bilateral). One of his parents or possibly one or more of his
siblings were similarly affected (see Fig. 4.3).

This proves that the inquirer has the hereditary, dominant
form of the disease. Each of his children, therefore, runs a
40% risk (1 : 1 ratio in the dominant mode of inheritance and
80% penetrance) of inheriting retinablastoma. In our opinion, this constitutes grounds for discouraging propagation.

The same reasoning applies if the parents and siblings are
unaffected but close relatives (such as grandparents, aunts,
uncles, etc.) have suffered from it. Such a situation would
mean that the dominant form is present but, for some reason,
did not manifest itself in one or several of the heterozygotes.

(b) Let us suppose that the inquirer himself is normal but
that several of his immediate relatives are affected; for instance, one of his parents and one of his siblings (see Fig. 4.4).

In this situation, two possibilities exist: either the proband
inherited the normal allele from his affected parent, or he

FIGURE 4.3. Sample genetic situation in cases of retinoblastoma.
Question:

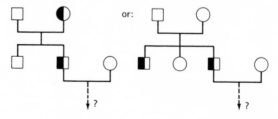

Answer:
The risk for every child = 40%

possesses a retinoblastoma gene which has not manifested itself. The former possibility exists with a 50% probability, the latter with a 10% probability for all the children of a trait bearer. Consequently, the proband has a chance of 50/50 + 10 = 50/60 = 83.3% of being free of the retinoblastoma gene. Should this be the case, all his children will be normal. If he is heterozygous, a 16.7% probability, then 40% of his children will be affected, a sum total risk of 6.52% for each of his children. This risk is not sufficiently high, in our opinion, to categorically advise against children, although it is a reason to keep any children under close medical surveillance until the manifestation period has passed.

The more normal children the inquirer has already produced, the better the chances that all further children will be normal. The minute that one of his children manifests the disease, the situation defines itself and we know that each succeeding child will manifest the disease with a 40% probability.

2. Let us now consider the counseling for the sporadic cases where there are no other affected family members: (a) The inquirer himself suffered from unilateral retinoblastoma. There are no other cases in the family and he would like to know the risk involved for his children (see Fig. 4.5).

From the general information at the beginning of this discussion we know that only 15 to 20% of the sporadic unilateral cases are dominant new mutations whose children run a 40% risk. The other 80% suffer from a nonhereditary form.

FIGURE 4.4. Sample genetic situation in cases of retinoblastoma.

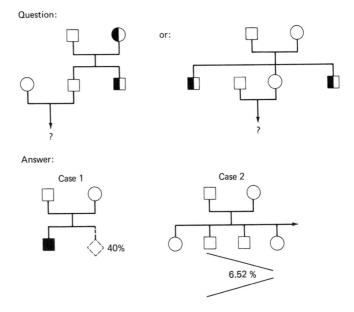

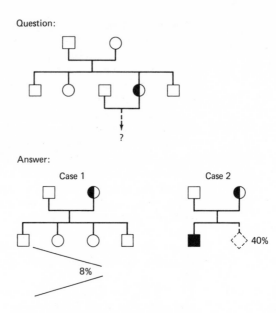

FIGURE 4.5. Sample genetic situation in cases of retinoblastoma.

Their children are perfectly normal. Since we cannot, as yet, distinguish the hereditary from the nonhereditary form, there remains a 6 to 8% risk that the proband will have an affected child. The risk involved is not big enough to advise against children, but medical surveillance of all children, at least until the danger age has passed, should be urgently recommended.

As usual, every normal child born to the family increases the probability that the proband belongs to the group suffering from the nonhereditary form of the disease. Therefore, the probability for further normal children increases proportionally. But the first affected child proves the contrary. The parent then definitely belongs to the group of dominant new mutations and future children again run that frightening 40% risk.

(b) The inquirer suffered from bilateral retinoblastoma but there are no further cases in the family (see Fig. 4.6).

All sporadic bilateral cases must be considered as dominant new mutations. This results in a 40% risk or every child. The patient should be urgently discouraged from propagating himself.

(c) We will now consider a frequent occurrence in practical counseling. The inquirer and all his relatives are unaffected but a child suffering from retinoblastoma has been born. The parents want to know the risk involved in having further children (see Fig. 4.7).

Question: Answer:

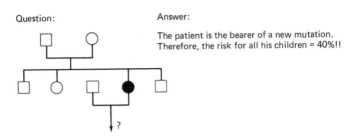

The patient is the bearer of a new mutation.
Therefore, the risk for all his children = 40%!!

FIGURE 4.6. Sample genetic situation in cases of retinoblastoma.

Question: Answer:

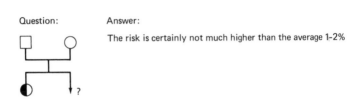

The risk is certainly not much higher than the average 1-2%

FIGURE 4.7. Sample genetic situation in cases of retinoblastoma.

In all probability, the case is either a new mutation or a nonhereditary defect. In both cases, it is highly improbable that further children will manifest the defect. On the other hand, there is a remote possibility that one of the parents carries the defective gene, but it did not manifest itself. This would once again mean a 40% risk for all future children. But, and this is to be expected, experience shows that this possibility is very remote indeed. According to Kaelin (1955; cited by Vogel, 1967), among 959 siblings of sporadic cases only 13 were affected (1.36%). The objection that it was a selected series and therefore resulted in very optimistic figures has been raised against Kaelin's statistics, but a more recent random series, undertaken in Holland, arrived at more or less the same results. Of 887 junior siblings of sporadic cases only 10 (1.13%) were affected, figures which correspond to Kaelin's estimate. Therefore, this risk is virtually negligible and no reason to advise against more children. As a reasonable precaution, however, later children should have regular eye examinations.

It is generally advisable to consider separately the risk for later siblings of unilateral and bilateral cases. Risk figures are somewhat (not much) higher for siblings of bilateral sporadic cases.

3. As a final situation, let us consider the problem of the normal brother or sister of a sporadic retinoblastoma case, who wishes to know the risk involved for his or her future children.

In such a case, there is a high degree of probability that both the inquirer and his children will be free of the retinoblastoma gene. The possibility that the gene is present but did not manifest itself either in him or his parents and can therefore affect his children is again very remote; no reason to advise against children. A group that examined 90 children of the siblings of 42 sporadic cases (28 unilateral, 14 bilateral) in respect to this possibility discovered only one affected child. Although there is no reason to advise against children, regular eye examinations for them should be strongly recommended.

5 The Autosomal Recessive Mode of Inheritance and Tests for the Detection of Heterozygotes

Compared to the problems presented by the autosomal recessive mode of inheritance, the autosomal dominant mode seems simple. Apart from very rare new mutations, the autosomal recessive mode presents one with the progeny of ostensibly normal parents who are heterozygous for the gene in question; i.e., they carry only one defective gene and the normal allele with its "healthy" information prevents the defect from manifesting itself. Figure 5.1 is a diagram of the typical situation.

It follows logically that every child from such a union has a 25% chance of inheriting two defective genes and therefore being homozygous and sick. The probability is 25% + 25% = 50% that the children will be, like the parents, heterozygous gene bearers. There remains the 25% chance that a child will inherit two normal genes and be homozygous for the normal allele; it will then be unable to pass on the defects. On the average, the ratio of normal to defective in such families is

FIGURE 5.1

The most typical mating pattern in the autosomal recessive mode of inheritance.

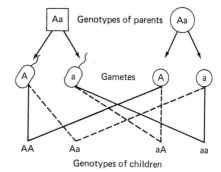

1 : 3. Once again, in this discussion the pattern of heredity and the manifestation probability are independent of sex. Among the relatives of affected individuals, further sufferers are to be expected primarily among their siblings who are also subject to the 25% homozygosity risk.

The size of the family unit has steadily decreased in industrial societies. Because each family has comparatively few children, it often seems *as if the sufferers of an autosomal-recessive defect were sporadic cases.* They tend to be the only affected member in their own family, and sometimes in the entire kinship; yet their disease is definitely hereditary. Therefore, with this mode of inheritance it is an error to conclude that the anomaly is not hereditary simply because there are no other cases in the family.

A simple example would be a series of two-children families with heterozygous parents. In only 1 in 16 families will both children be affected. In 6 cases, one child will be (sporadically) affected. According to the statistical laws of probability, in 9 families of the 16 no one will actually manifest the disease (see Fig. 5.2). This result is derived from the binomial distribution.

The example demonstrates clearly once more that *probable inheritance risks are only probability calculations.* A specific situation in a small family might deviate considerably from the norm. Furthermore, the example shows that for families with only one affected child, the defective to normal ratio is no longer 1 : 3; since all the parents whose children are only "accidentally" normal are never even considered as heterozygous, the frequency of actually affected individuals is much higher. For calculating the segregation ratios, this ascertainment bias can be corrected in order to arrive at more accurate figures.

The pathological gene can be passed on unnoticed from generation to generation in the autosomal-recessive mode of inheritance. Only the accidental union of two people who are

FIGURE 5.2. Expectancy ratio for sibships with two, one, and no sick members, given an autosomal-recessive mode of inheritance and two-child families with heterozygous parents (Aa × Aa).

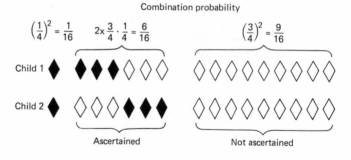

Combination probability

$$\left(\frac{1}{4}\right)^2 = \frac{1}{16} \qquad 2 \times \frac{3}{4} \cdot \frac{1}{4} = \frac{6}{16} \qquad \left(\frac{3}{4}\right)^2 = \frac{9}{16}$$

Child 1

Child 2

Ascertained   Not ascertained

both heterozygous for the same defective gene raises the 25%
probability that a child of theirs will be homozygous for that
particular gene and will therefore manifest the anomaly.

The rarer a gene in the population, the smaller the probability that the marriage partners will both have the same defective gene (to be exact, the probability equals the square of
the heterozygote frequency in the population). In a consanguinous marriage, however, the probability that both parties
have received the defective gene through some common
ancestor depends solely upon how closely the two are related.
Consequently, the rarer the gene, the rarer will be the accidental union of heterozygotes; it follows that a good part of
the total heterozygous unions will be marriages among relatives. We will deal with the problems raised by consanguinous
marriages later. At this point, the fact is only mentioned in
order to explain why, in general, individuals suffering from a
very rare genetic anomaly tend to stem from consanguinous
unions more often than sheer coincidence would permit.
*Should a patient whose disease has been clinically diagnosed
as hereditary have related parents, this fact strongly indicates
an autosomal recessive mode of inheritance.* This becomes
almost a certainty if the siblings are affected as well. The converse, on the other hand, is not valid. The fact that the parents
are not related does not exclude an autosomal recessive mode
of inheritance.

In genetic family counseling, one of the recurrent questions is the inquiry as to the probability that an individual who
has affected siblings is himself heterozygous for the defective
gene. Let us assume that the clinical diagnosis has been established beyond reasonable doubt, and that the defect is
hereditary and autosomal recessive, as for instance in a case
of phenylketonuria (Følling's disease). There are no other
cases within the family. Under these circumstances, the question is easily answered. The probability calculation for heterozygosity of the normal relatives, merely on the basis of common ancestry, is shown in the model pedigree of Fig. 5.3.

Of course, the values given in the diagram in Fig. 5.3 are
open to modification depending upon circumstances. If the
parents of the patient are first cousins, it is very likely that
the grandparents—who were siblings—were the gene carriers.
For the grandparents, in such a case, the probability of being
heterozygous will be greater than 50%; it approaches 100%.
Relatives who trace their ancestry to this line are correspondingly more "endangered." For the spouse of the suspect
grandparent, the risk becomes proportionately smaller and
approaches the values of the heterozygote frequency in the
population. Again, values will have to be adjusted for relatives
who trace their common ancestry to this single grandparent.
Apart from such situation variations, one must, of course, add
to the given values the general population probability figures,

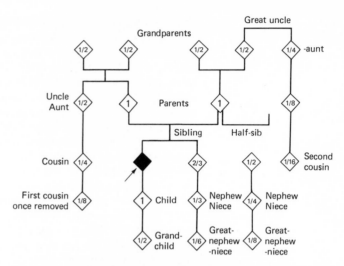

FIGURE 5.3. Probability figures for heterozygosity of relatives of a homozygote with an autosomal-recessive defect. (The sex of family members is not recorded since it makes no difference. For the sake of clarity, normal unrelated spouses have been omitted.) Values for further degrees of relationship can easily be deduced. It is simply a matter of tracing the ancestry in the most direct line and calculating that the chance of inheriting any specific gene from either parent by any child is 50%. The slightly different values for siblings of affected individuals are based on the fact that one group of children (the sick ones) has been excluded from the calculations (see Fig. 5.1).

i.e., those that estimate the chances that anyone might possess the gene in question by sheer accident.

The basis for this calculation lies in the estimated gene frequency figures for the population and in an assumption of "genetic equilibrium" for any gene. The genotype frequency is thereupon calculated according to the Hardy–Weinberg formula:

$$p^2 + 2pq + q^2 = 1 \quad \text{and} \quad p + q = 1.$$

p and q refer to the frequencies of the normal and the defective allels, p^2 and q^2 to the homozygote frequency, and $2pq$ to the heterozygote frequency. For phenylketonuria, for instance, the homozygote frequency (q^2) equals 0.0001 of the gene frequency (q) 0.01, and the heterozygote frequency ($2pq$) equals $2 \times 0.99 \times 0.01 = 0.0198$, i.e., approximately 1:50.[1]

[1] The situation for phenylketonuria is complicated since genetic heterogeneity apparently exists for the hyperphenylalaninemia symptom, i.e., the symptom may be caused by other genes as well. Apart from Følling's

In the discussion concerning the autosomal-dominant mode of inheritance, it was already pointed out that the categories of "recessive" and "dominant" represent oversimplifications whose definitions apply exactly only in extreme (textbook) cases. Therefore it comes as no surprise that, with many diseases of the autosomal-recessive category, a careful examination of the heterozygotes will show distinct if minor variations from the norm. Strictly speaking, one should thereupon once more discuss everything in terms of an intermediary mode of inheritance, but this would unnecessarily complicate matters. Thus, it has become common usage to speak of an autosomal-recessive mode of inheritance with recognizable heterozygosity. In some cases, a careful physical examination will reveal microsymptoms that indicate the presence of the defective gene in a single dose. In general, however, this is not possible and such proof requires very specialized test methods. Recently, a great deal of effort has been devoted to the development and systematization of these heterozygote detection tests.

The greatest success to date has been in the area of hereditary metabolic disturbances. These results are achieved either through refined test methods for analyzing the normal condition of the body or by overloading the critical metabolic pathways, a method that will frequently produce a variant reaction pattern in heterozygotes. Recently, further test methods, including histochemical and biochemical studies of cultured fibroblasts, have been developed. The reliability of such tests is established by comparing the results from a sample of known heterozygotes (such as "normal" parents of affected children) with those of a group of "normals."

Let us look at a relatively frequent situation as an example: The normal brother of a patient who is mentally defective due to phenylketonuria wants to marry and wishes to know whether he can responsibly enter into a marriage; also, whether he himself will pass on the gene and with what degree of risk for his children.

From our knowledge of the mode of inheritance of phenylketonuria, we can deduce (see Figs. 5.1 and 5.3) that the proband inherited the defective gene from one of his parents with a 2/3 probability. In the manner already discussed, we can calculate the prospective spouse's chances of being heterozygous for the gene. These two figures would then enable us to calculate the risk that the children will be homozygous for the defective gene. With many diseases subject to

disease, there exists a benign hyperphenylalaninemia. In all probability, the phenylketonuria frequency figures will soon be adjusted. These facts are not given due consideration at this point, first because final results are still lacking and second because the figures were employed primarily in order to demonstrate the calculation procedure.

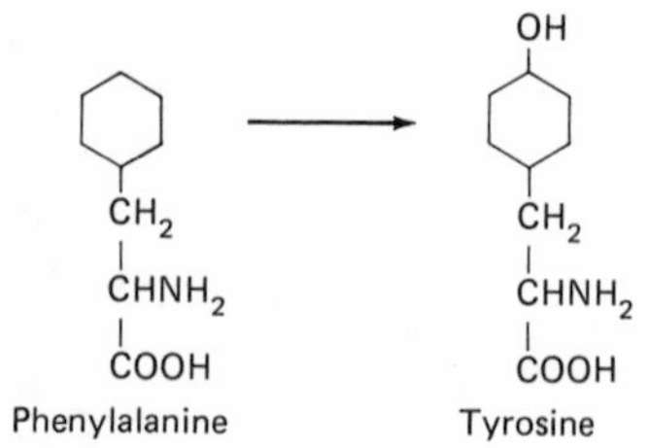

FIGURE 5.4

Enzyme defect in phenylketonuria: the catabolism of
phenylalanine into tyrosine is disrupted.

Phenylalanine → Tyrosine

this mode of inheritance, this is about all that can be done.
With very rare diseases, one can only recommend that the
individual in question should not marry a relative and that he
make sure that his prospective partner's family has no similarly affected members. If these last two conditions are met,
the chance that the children will be heterozygous is a little
above 1/3 and, although the risk of homozygosity for the
children will be higher than for the average population, it
will still be very small. To be more specific, in this case the
calculation would be $2/3 \times 1/50 = 1/75$ (see page 40) for
the probability that both parents are heterozygous (against the
average population probability of $1/50 \times 1/50 = 1/2500$).

Since the chance that the child will be homozygous for the
defective gene, should both parents be heterozygous, would
amount to 1/4, the combined probability would be $1/4 \times
1/75 = 1/300$. Granted, the risk is 33 times greater than the
risk for children of "unbiased" parents (1 in 10,000) but the
chance is still so small that negative counsel is unnecessary.

It so happens that in the case of phenylketonuria we can
be even more exact. The disease is based on an enzyme defect which inhibits the normal catabolism of phenylalanine
into tyrosine (Fig. 5-4).

The interference with the development of the brain depends upon the accumulation of phenylalanine and other abnormal metabolites resulting from this. Consequently, there is
a reduction in the patient's tyrosine concentration. The patient lacks the functioning enzyme, phenylalanine hydroxy-
lase, and experiments have shown that this enzyme is also
present in less than normal amounts in the systems of heterozygotes. Thus, when fasting, the mean concentration of phenylalanine in the serum of heterozygotes is slightly heightened.
The trouble is that the variation within the two classes (homozygote, heterozygote) is so great that a clear distinction between them is impossible (see Fig. 5.5).

This problem can be overcome by subjecting the patient's
system to a standard dose of L-phenylalanine and examining
the phenylalanine concentration in the plasma at set intervals.
Thus, the distribution becomes clearly bimodal. Apart from
the greater increase of the phenylalanine content in the

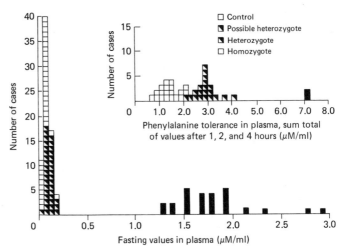

FIGURE 5.5. Outer graph: Phenylalanine concentration (mg-%) in the plasma of phenylketonurics, genetically established heterozygotes, and clinical "normals" (control persons). (Values for fasting without additional phenylalanine loading.) Inner graph: Phenylalanine content of plasma in the three above-mentioned groups after loading the system with 2 mmol L-phenylalanine/kg body weight; sum total values after one, two, and four hours in μM-ml.

After Jervis (cited in Linneweh, 1964)

heterozygote's plasma, there is the corresponding low in his tyrosine concentration (Fig. 5.6) compared to the norm. The test results can be made even more clearly distinctive by using a phenylalanine/tyrosine concentration ratio.

With the aid of these tests it becomes possible to more or less define the genotype of the proband. For about 20% of

(Text continues on page 51.)

FIGURE 5.6

Tyrosine concentration (mg-%) in the plasma of phenylketonurics, heterozygotes, and control persons in the phenylalanine tolerance test (2 mmol L-phenylalanine/kg body weight.

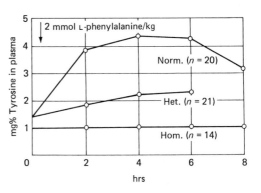

After Jervis (cited in Linneweh, 1964)

Table 5.1 Detection of Heterozygotes in Autosomal-Recessive Conditions

Condition	Abnormality in heterozygote	Reference
By direct measurement	*Red blood cells*	
Hemoglobinopathies	Variation in isoelectric point	Beet, E. A.: *Ann. Eugen., 14:* 279 (1949).
		Neel, J. V.: *Science, 110:* 64 (1949).
		Pauling, L., *et al.*: *Science, 110:* 543 (1949).
α-thalassemia	↑ Hb A$_2$	Kunkel, H. G., *et al.*: *J. Clin. Invest., 36:* 1615 (1957).
β-thalassemia	Hb Barts (γ4) in infancy	Weatherall, D. J.: *Brit. J. Haemat., 9:*265 (1963).
Argininosuccinic aciduria	↓ argininosuccinase	Tomlinson, S., *et al.*: *Clin. Sci., 26:*261 (1964).
Galactokinase deficiency	↓ galactokinase	Gitzelmann, R.: *Ped. Res., 1:* 14 (1967).
Galactosemia	↓ gal-1-P uridyl transferase (50% normal)	Hsia, D. Y-Y., *et al.*: *Nature, 182:*1389 (1958).
		Bretthauer, R. K., *et al.*: *Proc. Nat. Acad. Sci., 45:* 328 (1959).
		Kirkman, H. M., *et al.*: *Ann. Hum. Genet., 23:* 117 (1959).
Duarte variant	↓ gal-1-P uridyl transferase (75% normal)	Beutler, E.: personal communication.
		Mellman, W. J., *et al.*: *Ann. Hum. Genet., 32:*1 (1968).
Glycogen storage disease VI (hepatic phosphorylase deficiency)	↑ glycogen	Wallis, P. G., *et al.*: *Amer. J. Dis. Chid., 111:*278 (1966).
Increased glucose-6-phosphate dehydrogenase	↑ G-6-PD	Dearn, R. J.: *J. Lab. Clin. Med., 68:* 560 (1966).
6-phosphogluconic dehydrogenase deficiency	↓ 6-P-GD in Dalston variant (75% normal)	Parr, C. W., *et al.*: *Ann. Hum. Genet., 30:*339 (1967).
Pyruvate kinase deficiency	↓ PK	Tanaka, K. R., *et al.*: *Blood, 19:*267 (1962).
Triosephosphate isomerase deficiency	↓ TPI	Schneider, A. S., *et al.*: *Hereditary Disorders of Erythrocyte Metabolism* (E. Beutler, ed.) New York, Grune & Stratton, 1968, p. 265.
Hexokinase deficiency	↓ hexokinase	Valentie, W. N., *et al.*: *New Eng. J. Med., 276:*1 (1967).

Condition	Marker	Reference
Methemoglobinemia, congenital	↓ NADP diaphorase	Scott, E. M.: *J. Clin. Invest.*, 39: 1176 (1960).
Acatalasemia (Japanese variant)	↓ catalase	Nishimura, E. T., et al.: *Science*, 130:333 (1959).
Acatalasemia (Swiss variant)	↓ catalase	Aebi, H., et al.: *Enz. Biol. Clin.*, 2:1 (1962).
Orotic aciduria	↓ orotidylic decarboxylase	Fallon, H. J., et al.: *New Eng. J. Med.*, 270:878 (1964).
Glycogen synthetase deficiency	↓ tolerance to glucose*	Lewis, G. M., et al.: *Arch. Dis. Child.*, 38:40 (1963).

White blood cells

Condition	Marker	Reference
Maple syrup urine disease	leucine-1-^{14}C → ^{14}CO$_2$	Dancis, J., et al.: *J. Pediat.*, 66:595 (1965).
Intermittent branched-chain ketonuria	↓ isovaleric-1-^{14}C → ^{14}CO$_2$	Dancis, J., et al.: *New Eng. J. Med.*, 276:84 (1967).
Galactosemia	↓ gal-1-P uridyl transferase	Inouye, T., et al.: *Clin. Chem. Acta*, 19:169 (1968).
		Mellman, W.J., et al.: *J. Lab. Clin. Med.*, 66:980 (1965).
Duarte variant	↓ gal-1-P uridyl transferase	Beutler, E., et al.: *J. Lab. Clin. Med.*, 68:646 (1966).
Glycogen storage disease II (Pompe's disease)	↓ α-glucosidase	Nitowsky, H. M., et al.: *J. Lab. Clin. Med.*, 69: 472 (1967).
Glycogen storage disease III (debrancher deficiency)	↓ amylo-1,6-glucosidase	Chayoth, R., et al.: *Israel J. Med. Sci.*, 3:422 (1967).
Triose phosphate isomerase deficiency	↓ TPI	Williams, H. E., et al.: *J. Clin. Invest.*, 42:656 (1963).
		Schneider, A. S., et al.: *Hereditary Disorders of Erythrocyte Metabolism* (E. Beutler, ed.) New York, Grune & Stratton, 1968, p. 265.
Orotic aciduria	↓ orotidylic aciduria	Smith, L. H., et al.: *The Metabolic Basis of Inherited Disease* (J. B. Stanbury, et al., ed.) New York, McGraw–Hill, 1966, p. 739.
Cystinosis	↑ cystine	Schneider, J. A. et al.: *Science*, 157:1321 (1967).

Table 5.1 Detection of Heterozygotes in Autosomal-Recessive Conditions (continued)

Condition	Abnormality in heterozygote	Reference
Batten-Spielmeyer-Vogt syndrome	↑ abnormal granulation	Zeman, W., et al.: *Inborn Disorders of Sphingo-lipid Metabolism* (S. M. Aronson, et al., ed.) New York, Pergamon Press, 1967, p. 475.
Chediak-Higashi syndrome	↑ inclusions	Kritzler, R. A., et al.: *Amer. J. Med.* 36:583 (1964).
	Plasma or serum	
PTA deficiency (factor XI)	↓ PTA	Rapaport, S. I., et al.: *Blood, 18*:149 (1961).
Hageman deficiency (factor XII)	↓ correction of Hageman deficiency	Ratnoff, O. D., et al.: *J. Lab. Clin. Med., 59*:980 (1962).
Labile factor deficiency (factor V)	↓ labile factor	Kingsley, C. S.: *Quart. J. Med., 23*: 323 (1954).
Stuart-Prower deficiency (factor X)	↑ prothrombin time	Graham, J. B., et al.: *J. Clin. Invest., 36*:497 (1957).
Fibrin stabilizing factor deficiency (factor XIII)	↓ FSF	Atencio, A., et al.: *Clin. Res.*, in press
Afibrinogenemia (factor I)	↓ fibrinogen	Frick, P. G., et al.: *Pediatrics, 13*:44 (1954).
Hypophosphatasia	↓ alkaline phosphatase	Harris, H., et al.: *Ann. Hum. Genet., 23*:421 (1959).
Fat-induced hyperlipoproteinemia	↓ lipoprotein lipase	Havel, R. J., et al.: *J. Clin. Invest., 39*:1777 (1960).
Tangier disease	↓ high density lipoprotein	Fredrickson, D. S.: *J. Clin. Invest., 43*: 228 (1964).
A-β-lipoproteinemia	↓ β-lipoprotein	Salt, H. B., et al.: *Lancet, 2*:325 (1960).
Tay-Sachs disease	↓ F-1-P aldolase	Volk, B. W., et al.: *Amer. J. Med., 36*:481 (1964).
Hemochromatosis	↑ iron	Debre, R., et al.: *Ann. Hum. Genet., 23*:16 (1958).
Prothrombin deficiency (factor II)	↑ prothrombin time[a]	Quick, A. J., et al.: *Lancet, 1*:173 (1962).
Stable factor deficiency (factor VII)	↑ prothrombin time[a]	Dische, F. E., et al.: *Acta Haemat., 21*:257 (1959).

Condition	Finding	Reference
Hyperglycinemia	↑ glycine[a]	Schreier, K., et al.: German Med. Monthly, 9: 437 (1964).
Urine		
Argininosuccinic aciduria	↑ argininosuccinic acid	Corgell, M. E., et al.: Biochem. Biophys. Res. Comm., 14: 307 (1964).
Cystathionuria	↑ cystathionine	Frimpter, G. W., et al.: New Eng. J. Med., 268: 33 (1963).
Cystinuria (type II)	↑ arginine	Crawhall, J. C., et al.: Ann. Hum. Genet., 29:257 (1966).
Tissue		
Homocystinuria	↓ liver cystathionine synthetase	Finkelstein, J. D., et al.: Science, 146:785 (1964).
Crigler-Najjar syndrome	↓ liver glucuronyl transferase	Arias, I. M.: J. Clin. Invest., 41: 2233 (1962).
Histidinemia	↓ skin histidase	Ladu, B. N., et al.: Pediatrics, 32:216 (1963).
Glycogen storage disease I (Von Gierke's disease)	↓ intestinal glucose-6-phosphatase	Field, J. B., et al.: J. Clin. Invest., 44:1240 (1965).
Disaccharidase intolerance	↓ intestinal sucrase, maltase, isomaltase	Prader, A., et al.: Ann. Rev. Med., 16:345 (1965).
Cretinism with goiter	thyroid goiter	Stanbury, J. B., et al.: Lancet, 1:1162 (1960).
Female, in X-linked recessive conditions, by direct measurement		
Red blood cells		
Glucose-6-phosphate dehydrogenase deficiency	↓ G-6-PD	Childs, B., et al.: Bull. John Hop. Hosp., 102:21 (1958).
White blood cells		
	↓ G-6-PD	Ramot, B., et al.: J. Clin. Invest., 38:2234 (1959).
Plasma or serum		
AHG deficiency (classial hemophilia) (fator VIII)	↓ AHG	Rapaport, S. I., et al.: Amer. J. Clin. Invest., 39: 1619 (1960).

Table 5.1 Detection of Heterozygotes in Autosomal-Recessive Conditions (continued)

Condition	Abnormality in heterozygote	Reference
PTC deficiency (Christmas disease) (factor IX)	↓ PTC	Simpson, N. E., et al.: Brit. J. Haemat., 8:191 (1962).
X-linked Duchenne muscular dystrophy	↑ CPK,[a] change LDH isoenzyme[a]	Dreyfus, J. C., et al.: Biochemistry of Hereditary Myopathies, Springfield, Ill., Charles C. Thomas, 1962. Emery, A. E. H.: Nature, 201: 1044 (1964).
Urine		
Nephrogenic diabetes insipidus	↓ Specific gravity	Carter, C., el al.: Lancet, 2: 1069 (1956).
Tissues		
Fabry's disease	↓ Intestinal ceramidetrihexosidase	Brady, R. O. et al.: New Eng. J. Med., 276: 1163 (1967).
X-linked Duchenne muscular dystrophy	Muscle cells divided into two groups	Pearson, C. M., et al.: Proc. Nat. Acad. Sci., 50: 29 (1963).
Using cell cultures	*Direct measurement in fibroblasts*	
Galactosemia	↓ gal-1-P uridyl transferase	Krooth, R. S., et al.: J. Exp. Med., 113: 1115
Glycogen storage disease II (Pompe's disease)	↓ α-glusocidase	Nitowsky, H. M., et al.: J. Lab. Clin. Med., 69: 472 (1967).
Acatalasemia (Japanese variant)	↓ catalase	Krooth, R. S. et al.: J. Exp. Med., 115: 313 (1962).
Orotic aciduria	↓ orotidylic decarboxylase	Krooth, R. S.:Quart. Biol., 29: 189 (1964).
Cystinosis	↑ cystine	Schneider, J. A., et al.: Biochem. Biophys. Res. Comm., 29: 527 (1967).
	Metachromasia in fibroblasts	
Cystic fibrosis of pancreas	Present in heterozygotes	Danes, B. S., et al.: Lancet, 1: 241 (1967).

Condition	Detection	Reference
Gaucher's disease	Present in heterozygotes	Danes, B. S., et al.: Lancet, 1: 1061 (1968).
Batten-Spielmeyer-Vogt syndrome	Present in heterozygotes	Danes, B. S., et al.: Science, 161: 1347 (1968).
Hurler's syndrome	Present in heterozygotes	Danes, B. S., et al.: Lancet, 2: 65 (1967).
Mucopolysaccharidosis	Present in heterozygotes	Danes, B. S., et al.: Lancet, 2:855 (1968).
Lipomucopolysaccharidosis	Present in heterozygotes	Matalon, R., et al.: Proc. Nat. Acad. Sci., 59: 1097 (1968).
Hurler's syndrome variant	Present in heterozygotes	Leroy, J. G., et al.: Science, 157:804 (1967).
Chediak-Higashi syndrome	Present in heterozygotes	Danes, B. S., et al.: J. Exp. Med., 126:509 (1967).
Cystic fibrosis of pancreas	*Metachromasia in white blood cells* Present in heterozygotes	Geisler, M., et al.: ???? Kinderheilk, 112:133 (1972).
Female, in X-linked recessive conditions, using cloning technique with cell cultures		
Glucose-6-phosphate dehydrogenase	Two populations with G-6-PD$^+$ and G-6-PD$^-$ cells	Davidson, R. G., et al.: Proc. Nat. Acad. Sci., 50:481 (1963).
Lesch-Nyhan syndrome	Two populations with HGPRT$^+$ and HGPRT$^-$ cells	Migeon, B. R., et al.: Science, 160: 425 (1968).
Hunter's syndrome	Two populations with metachromatic$^+$ and metachromatic$^-$ cells	Danes, B. S., et al.: Lancet, 2:65 (1967).
Fetal granulomatosis of childhood	Two populations with difference in phagocytosis/histochemical test	Windhorst, D. B. et al.: Lancet, 1:737 (1967).
Wilson's disease (^{64}Cu by mouth)[b]	↑ ^{64}Cu (48 h)/ ^{64}Cu (1-2 h) (serum)	Sternlieb, I., et al.: J. Clin. Invest., 40:707 (1961).
Phenylketonuria (Phenylalanine)	↑ phenylalanine (serum)	Hsia, D. Y-Y., et al.: Nature, 178:1239 (1956).
Cystathioninuria (Methione)	↑ cystathionine (urine)	Mongeau, J. G., et al.: J. Pediat, 69:1113 (1966).
Hyperlysinemia (Lysine)	↑ lysine (serum)	Ghadimi, H., et al.: New Eng. J. Med., 273:724 (1965).
Hypersarcosinemia (Sarcosine)	↑ sarcosine (urine)	Gerritsen, T., et al.: Pediatrics, 36:882 (1965).

Table 5.1 Detection of Heterozygotes in Autosomal-Recessive Conditions (continued)

Condition	Abnormality in heterozygote	Reference
Pentosuria (D-glucuronolactone)	↑ L-xylulose (serum) (urine)	Freedberg, I. M., et al.: Biochem. Biophys. Res. Comm., 1: 328 (1959).
Cretinism with goiter; deiodinase defect (^{131}I-labeled di-iodotyrosine)	↑ labeled substance (urine)	Stanbury, J. B., et al.: J. Clin. Endocr., 16:848 (1956).
Crigler-Najjar syndrome (Salicylate)	↓ glucuronic acid conjugation (urine)	Childs, B., et al.: Pediatrics, 23:903 (1959).
Hyperoxaluria (^{14}C-carboxyl-labeled glyoxylate)	↓ utilization of labeled material (urine)	Frederick, E. W., et al.: New Eng. J. Med., 269: 821 (1963).
Tyrosinemia (Phenylalanine)	↑ Million-reacting substance (urine)	Gentz, J., et al.: Amer. J. Dis. Child, 113: 31 (1967).
Hyperglycinemia (Glycine)	↑ glycine (serum)[a]	Tada, K., et al.: Tohoku J. Exp. Med., 85: 105 (1965).
Hydroxykynureninuria (Tryptophan)	↑ xanthurenic acid (urine)[a]	Komrower, G. M., et al.: Arch. Dis. Child., 39: 250 (1964).
Diabetes mellitus (Cortisone-glucose)	abnormal glucose tolerance tests[a]	Fajans, S. S., et al.: Diabetes, 3: 269 (1954).

[a]Requires further study and confirmation.
[b]Loading material.
Source: Adapted from Hsia, D. Y.-Y.: Med. Clin. North Amer., 53: 857 (1969).

those heterozygous for the phenylketonuria gene, however, it will virtually be impossible to find values that differ markedly from those of normal homozygotes. It is therefore possible to say with almost absolute certainty that a person is heterozygous, but the converse, that he is free of the defective gene, can only be stated with an 80% probability.

In general, the situation with other hereditary diseases is far more uncertain. Though it may be possible to delimit the group of heterozygotes quite well, a definite statement concerning the status of a particular examined individual can only be made with reservations. Just the same, heterozygote tests and their results frequently do facilitate the ultimate counseling. The tests can also be used to improve the probability figures for the possibility that the heterozygote's potential spouse (of normal family, according to its pedigree) is not, by sheer chance, also heterozygous for the defective gene.

The aim of this type of research is, of course, to find ways and means of detecting heterozygotes. Genetic defects and diseases for which tests have been developed that allow us to establish heterozygosity are listed in Table 5.1, with an index of the more detailed literature for specific diseases. This list is growing steadily. An important recent development is the possibility of detecting enzyme defects in fibroblast cultures (Davidson, 1970).

At this point, the doctor as well as the patient is confronted with the following question: from the eugenic point of view, can a heterozygote for a serious genetic defect responsibly enter into any marriage? It is obvious that excluding all heterozygous carriers from propagation would lead to a reduction of the population frequency figures for any recessive defect. The trouble is that the number of heterozygotes who actually come for counseling is only a minute fraction of the total number of unknown heterozygotes in the population. With the rarer genetic defects and diseases, the fraction is so small that the exclusion of these few would not, even in a long-range view, significantly ameliorate the frequency figures. Counseling is directly and justifiably concerned with attempting to prevent marriages between heterozygotes in order to prevent the birth of sick children. Should the marriage already have taken place, we may advise against children, or further children. Should a child be conceived in spite of this, we urgently recommend close medical attention for the child in order to permit early diagnosis and therapy, where possible.

In conclusion, let us consider slightly rarer cases:

An individual suffering from a relatively minor genetic defect or disease may himself wish to marry. In this case, should the disease have an autosomal-recessive mode of inheritance, the individual in question is himself homozygous for the defective gene and all his children will be, at best, heterozy-

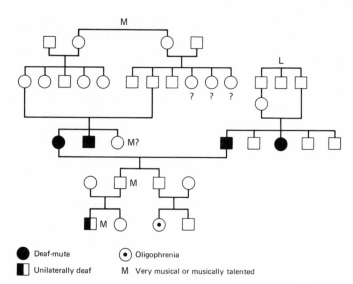

Deaf-mute   Oligophrenia
Unilaterally deaf   M   Very musical or musically talented

FIGURE 5.7. Pedigree proving genetic heterogeneity for deaf-mutism. Both parents derive from a consanguinous marriage, and yet the children are normal.

After Muehlmann (1930; cited in Vogel, 1961)

gotes. Moreover, there is the further possibility that his partner is heterozygous for the same gene. The probability of this, assuming that the partner comes from a normal family and is not related, equals the average heterozygote frequency in the population. This percentage multiplied by 1/2 will give the probability figures for affected children from this union. Should a sick child be born, it means that the partner is definitely heterozygous and every future child is subject to the 50% probability that it too will be affected.

A marriage between two homozygotes for the same defective gene can only result in sick children, since neither partner possesses a normal allele at this particular gene locus.

An apparent exception to this rule occurs (excluding the possibility of illegitimacy) if both parents have a clinically identical autosomal-recessive disease where the causal defect is traceable to different gene loci (heterogeneity, see p. H53). Muehlmann's pedigree for autosomal-recessive deaf-mutism offers an example (Fig. 5.7).

Example 5: At birth, the girl gave evidence of the typical Langdon Down syndrome (mongolism) symptoms: epicanthus, hypertelorism, hyperextensible joints, etc. Besides this, the university hospital diagnosed phenylketonuria. A chromosome analysis showed the typical G trisomy of the nondisjunction type (47 chromosomes; among the G-group chromosomes one small chromosome too many). The mother was aged 23 and the father 27 at the time of the birth.

The family pedigree (medical case history) showed that the parents were unrelated and that the preceding generation on either side was free of all "peculiarities." But a child of the same parents, born three years previously, had also manifested a case of phenylketonuria.

The combination of phenylketonuria and mongolism must be regarded as coincidental since further such cases are unknown to genetic literature. For the genetic prognosis, the phenylketonuria alone is important. Evidently, both parents are heterozygotes. Further children will manifest the disease with a 25% probability. Added to this is the approximately 1% risk (see Table 7.1) of mongolism. We strongly advised against any further children. A warning after the birth of the first child—had the family physician had the knowledge—might have prevented the conception of this girl.

With an as yet small but constantly increasing number of autosomal-recessive defects it is now possible to diagnose the condition during embryonic development. This means that the pregnancy can be interrupted if the diagnosis is positive (see Chapter 9 on prenatal diagnosis). This diagnostic field is rapidly expanding and the practicing physician should inquire whether such a diagnostic possibility exists for a given defect in a particular case.

Example 6: A young couple has already lost two children in infancy. The cause has been diagnosed as Pompe's disease, or glycogen-storage disease type 2. This defect is characterized by an α, 1, 4-glucosidase deficiency with an autosomal-recessive mode of inheritance. The deaths of the first two children coupled with the 25% risk for future progeny would have decided these parents against further children. However, this particular enzyme defect can be detected in amnion cells. The couple decided to risk a further pregnancy and an amniocentesis was carried out in the 14th week. Unfortunately, the cultivation of the amnion cells produced only very few cells, so that a clear diagnosis was not possible. The test was repeated, this time successfully. During the 20th week of the pregnancy the couple could be informed that this child was free from the defect, a diagnosis that was later confirmed by the birth of a healthy boy.[2]

According to McKusick (1975), there are approximately 950 known autosomal-recessive diseases.

[2] The amniocentesis and the cell culture were carried out by Dr. Berle and Dr. Passarge, respectively, both of Hamburg. The enzyme analysis was done by Dr. G. Hug of Cincinnati.

6 Sex-Linked Modes of Inheritance

The sex of the human being is genotypically determined. Male and female differ in that the male possesses an X and a Y chromosome whereas the female has two X chromosomes. Every fertile marriage therefore corresponds to the Mendelian backcross.

	Paternal gametes	
Maternal gametes	X	Y
X	¼ XX	¼ XY
X	¼ XX	¼ XY
Total	½ XX ♀	½ XY ♂

A gene located on one of the two sex chromosomes must necessarily show a totally different mode of inheritance from that of an autosomal gene. This mode of inheritance is easily deduced from the diagram illustrating the process of sex determination.

Empiric observation has, for all practical purposes, proved that there is no such thing as a Y-chromosomal mode of inheritance—with one possible and so far unimportant exception. Therefore we need only consider the X-chromosomal modes of inheritance, among which the X-chromosomal recessive mode is the one with the greatest practical importance.

The most frequent combinations of this mode of inheritance are as follows:

1. The mother is homozygous and normal (XX); the father is

hemizygous and affected (X′Y).[1] All sons of this union will be normal; they inherit the normal gene by way of the maternal X chromosome. All daughters, however, are heterozygous (X′X); the defective gene is located on the paternal X′ chromosome. Half the sons of these daughters will inherit the defective gene.

2. The mother is a heterozygous carrier (X′X), herself phenotypically normal. The father is normal (XY). In this case, half the sons will be affected (X′Y), whereas all the daughters will be normal. However, half the daughters will be heterozygous carriers (conductors).

3. Should an affected homozygous woman marry a normal man, all the sons will be affected, whereas all the daughters will be phenotypically normal conductors (carriers).

The remaining possible combinations are easily deduced. We will not go into them here because, in fact, they hardly ever occur in counseling practice.

The X-chromosomal recessive mode of inheritance is characterized by the fact that—especially with rare diseases— almost only men are affected. The path of inheritance, however, runs only via the normal daughters of sick fathers and half the normal sisters of sick men. This situation changes only if the brother's anomaly can be traced to a new mutation, in which case the sisters will not be conductors. What is even worse, all the daughters of affected fathers will be conductors.

This brief sketch of the mode of inheritance already indicates the obvious guidelines for family counseling. To take hemophilia A, a well-known genetic anomaly, as an example: Let us suppose that the daughter of a bleeder inquires as to the probability that her children will be affected. The answer is simple. The overall risk to all children is 25%, because there is a 50% probability for each child to be male, and if the child is a son, he again has a 50% risk of inheriting the defective gene from his mother, who must be heterozygous.

Conversely, the sons of bleeders will be normal. They can also be sure that they are not conductors (carriers) for the defective gene and that they will not pass it on to any of their offspring. In this case, a son can only be a bleeder should the mother prove accidentally heterozygous for the hemophilia gene, but as a rule this probability is negligible. Again, this rule does not apply should the marriage be consanguineous, i.e., if the mother and father are first cousins or otherwise closely related.

Let us suppose that the sister of a bleeder wishes to marry and inquires as to the degree of risk involved for her future children. The answer, theoretically, is very simple. The brother

[1] X′ indicates the chromosome carrying the defective gene, X the normal chromosome.

must, of necessity, have inherited the defective gene from his mother. The mother is therefore heterozygous and has also passed on the defective gene to half her daughters (average). The inquirer's chances of being heterozygous amount to 50%. If she did inherit the hemophilia gene, then 1 : 4 of her children will be affected (1/2 her sons). The probability figures for her children therefore total 1 : 8, with a 1 : 4 ratio for her sons.

In many cases, this general conclusion is regarded as sufficient and the matter is left here. If a woman has borne several healthy and unaffected sons, this additional information may be used to recalculate her risk of being heterozygous. If she were heterozygous, each son would have a 50% chance of being afflicted. With every healthy son, the chance of being homozygous and normal increases. The calculation is based on the Bayes theorem. The attempts to use the factor VIII activity in the plasma for differentiation between homozygous normal and heterozygous women have been unsuccessful in the past, since the variability of factor VIII activity has been very large in both groups, and extensive overlap has prohibited proper classification of single cases. Recently developed techniques using the ratio between amount of factor VIII antigenic material and factor VIII activity in the plasma have proved to be quite reliable in some pilot studies and will probably be standardized in the near future (Ratnoff and Bennett, 1973). At present, however, they are not yet really reliable. In any case, only results from laboratories with comprehensive experience should be used.

Special consideration should also be given to the question of whether or not the affected individual is a new mutant, a possibility that becomes very important if he is the only case within the closer degrees of kinship; i.e., if he is a sporadic case. The sporadic occurrence of hemophilia A and B as of other relatively frequent X-chromosomal genetic diseases, such as the Duchenne form of dystrophia musculorum progressiva, is not at all rare; it is much more frequent, in fact, than the textbook cases of pedigrees with massed familial incidence of a disease. Hence, the possibilities are twofold: First, the mother is a normal homozygote and the mutation occurred in the maternal germ cell. Should this be the case, the sisters of the patient have an almost 100% chance of being normal homozygotes who will produce normal children. Or the mother is a heterozygote; perhaps the mutation occurred in one of the germ cells of her parents, or her mother was already heterozygous. In the latter case, there is a 50% probabiilty that sisters of the patient will possess the defective gene.

The two possibilities are often very hard to differentiate. With hemophilia A, our present knowledge seems to indicate that the majority of new mutations occur in the male germ cells; e.g., those of the maternal grandfather of a patient. If this is correct, (nearly) all mothers of sporadic hemophiliacs would be heterozygotes, a hypothesis that seems to be confirmed by AHF test results. That means that a woman who has given birth to a son suffering from hemophilia A, will, with a 50% probability, produce further hemophilic sons—independent of whether there are other bleeders in the family or whether the child has the same or a different father.

The opposite seems to be true of muscular dystrophy, type Duchenne. Statistical research indicates that the majority of sporadic cases originate with a mutation in the maternal germ cell. The problem—whether or not a mother is heterozygous —will therefore have to be determined individually. The determination of the enzymes in the blood, especially the creatin phosphokinase (CPK), would help. Frequently, however, this examination does not decide the matter. Besides, in women older than 20 to 30, it becomes still more unreliable.

For the remaining less frequent X-chromosomal anomalies, there is little or no information concerning the occurrence of new mutations, despite the fact that this possibility is one that must always be considered. For some of these diseases, however, there are test methods that indicate heterozygosity—though, admittedly, with varying degrees of certitude.

The second sex-linked mode of inheritance is the X-chromosomal dominant one. This mode differs from the X-chromosomal recessive mode in that not only the hemizygotes (male) but also the heterozygotes (female) manifest the anomaly. Both men and women are affected, even when the anomaly is a rare one. All the sons of affected fathers are unaffected but all the daughters are trait bearers as well as half the sisters of the father. Among the children of the female patients there is a 1 : 1 segregation as in the autosomal-dominant mode of inheritance—i.e., independent of sex.

In brief, male patients must have inherited the trait from the mother; among their siblings there is a 1 : 1 segregation independent of sex. Female patients may have inherited the defective gene from either father or mother.

These facts alone serve to demonstrate that insufficient data may make it terribly difficult to differentiate between the X-chromosomal-dominant and the autosomal-dominant modes of inheritance.

The well-known anomalies subject to the X-chromosomal dominant mode of inheritance are Vitamin D resistant rickets with hypophosphatemia, some types of ectodermal anidrotic dysplasia, and genetic defects of the enzyme, glucose-6-phosphate dehydrogenase. To these, as well as to other examples, one rule applies: *When there is an X-chromosomal-dominant mode of inheritance, male patients are on the average more severely affected than their female counter-parts.*

The following rules for genetic family counseling can be deduced from these general criteria:

1. Male patients pass on the defective gene to all their daughters. On the average, these will suffer a lighter case of the anomaly.
2. Female patients will pass the defective gene to half their children, regardless of sex. As a rule, the sons will be more severely affected than the daughters.
3. In cases of complete dominance, individuals who are themselves phenotypically normal, regardless of their sex, will, with a probability approaching 100%, be free of the defective gene and have normal children.
4. In sporadic cases, a very careful examination is required in order to ensure that the symptoms, and the results of bio-chemical tests, are identical with the symptoms of ascer-tained genetic cases. This would exclude the possibility of a phenocopy. Thereupon one would have to verify that the parents are really free of microsymptoms. Should these conditions apply, then one can be almost certain that a new mutation occurred in one of the germ cells of one of the parents. For further children from this union, the risk of developing the anomaly is negligible. For any offspring of the new mutant, however, the above rules apply. In this respect, there is no difference; descendants of new mu-tants are subject to the same rules of inheritance as a family with a long history of affected members.

There is one rather special aspect of the X-chromosomal-dominant mode of inheritance. Some of these anomalies are prenatally lethal to all hemizygotes, whereas heterozygotes manifest phenotypical anomalies. In these cases, the defective gene is passed on to half the daughters of heterozygous mothers. Only normal sons are born; there are only affected females. These women may, but do not necessarily, show an increased tendency toward miscarriage.

This mode of inheritance was defined as a result of re-search with incontinentia pigmenti Bloch-Sulzberger, a skin disease with additional symptoms such as missing teeth (Lenz, 1961; for a detailed description, see Vogel and Dorn, 1964), and with the oro-facio-digital (OFD) syndrome, the combination of a median harelip and cleft palate with other cleavages in the oral area, and syndactyly characteristic of this condition (for details, see Fuhrmann et al., 1966).

The death of the hemizygous embryos results in considera-ble natural selection against the defective gene. Conse-quently, a high ratio of new mutations and sporadic cases among the sum total of affected individuals is only to be expected. However, in counseling the parents of a sporadic case, one must be extremely careful. With the OFD syndrome, the expressivity of the symptoms is highly variable. The traces of an incontinentia pigmenti that has run its course may sometimes be hardly, if at all, apparent in an adult woman. The mother must be very carefully examined. Despite these precautions, it may be virtually impossible, in a particular case, to distinguish whether one is confronted with a new mutation or a heterozygous mother. Should the latter be the case, there is a 1/2 probability of being affected for the next daughter. A history of miscarriages would corroborate the suspicion of heterozygosity.

The known sex-linked mutations number nearly 170 (McKusick, 1975).

7 Chromosome Aberrations

Down's Syndrome (Mongolism)

This syndrome is not only serious and well-known, it is also relatively frequent (approximately 1 : 500 to 1 : 600 births). For this reason, many parents of mongoloid children come for counseling and wish to know the risk involved in having further children. At the same time, this syndrome is an excellent example of a defect whose roots are so complex that no generally applicable formula for counseling can be given. It again illustrates how very carefully one must examine each individual case if one is to avoid major errors.

The following factors are the most important: (1) the age of the mother at the time of birth and (2) the cytogenetic facts.

AGE OF THE MOTHER

The probability of bearing a mongoloid child increases sharply with the age of the mother, for older women (above 40 or even 45) the probability is a multiple of that for women in their twenties or thirties. The probability also does not increase at a regular rate. It remains fairly static throughout the twenties and early thirties, thereafter increasing more and more every year. Considering the relative instead of the absolute frequency in relation to the mothers' age group (see Fig. 7.1), there seems to be a bimodal distribution. The left peak corresponds more or less to the distribution for the mother's age group in the general population, whereas the right peak appears with the considerably older group of mothers. The distribution indicates that there seems to be two types of groups. With the first type, the age of the mother is apparently unrelated to the cause, whereas it becomes the major factor with the second type. This hypothesis is con-

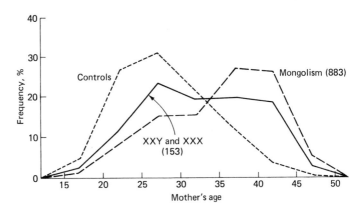

FIGURE 7.1. Age of the mother in cases of Down's syndrome and XXY types (Klinefelter) and XXX (Triple-X women) in comparison to the normal population (British data).

After Penrose (1967)

firmed upon studying the probability figures for the birth of further mongoloid children (Table 7.1).

The chances of a repetition of the misfortune for younger women who already have a child suffering from the syndrome increase sharply compared to others in the same age group, whereas the danger increases only negligibly compared to the average for older women with a mongoloid child. These facts suggest that there is such a thing as a constitutional disposition for producing such children which is found in a higher proportion of young women. According to more recent calculations (Mikkelsen and Stene, 1970), the recurrence risk of a 21-trisomy Down syndrome is 1 to 2% for mothers under 30; for women over 30, according to the same authors, the risk is the same as the population average. Absolutely speaking, the risk is about the same for all age groups, but considering the relative risk of bearing a mongoloid child within the same age group allows a different picture to emerge.

THE CYTOGENETIC FACTS

Counseling is, fortunately, no longer obliged to rely solely upon statistics. Chromosome analysis has given a much clearer picture.

As we know since 1959, mongolism is the result of one chromosome too many; one chromosome of group G, somewhat arbitrarily numbered 21, does not occur twice as is normal, but three times. This is described as a trisomy.

As a rule, trisomies occur as a result of nondisjunction of homologous chromosomes during one of the two meiotic divisions. This results in one germ cell having one chromo-

Table 7.1 Recurrence Risk after Birth of One Child with Down's Syndrome[a]

Karyotype of the child	Frequency among all cases with Down's syndrome	Karyotype of the mother	Karyotype of the father	Frequency of this constellation	Recurrence risk for further children
Free trisomy = 21 (47, XX, or XY, +21)[b]	95%	Normal	Normal	Most frequent constellation	1% (—2%)
		One-parent mosaic (supernumerary G chromosome in one cell line)	Normal	Rare	Uncertain, depending on type of the mosaic
Mosaic 46/47	1–2% (more frequent in atypical cases)	Normal	Normal		Probably 1%
Translocation trisomies	3%	(About 8% of all cases with mothers < 30 years of age; 1.5% of all cases with mothers > 30 years of age)			
Translocation D/G 46, XY or XX, —D, +t (DqGq)		Normal	Normal	⅔ of all cases with D/G translocation	
		Balanced translocation	Normal	2% of all cases with Down syndrome	10–12%
		Normal	Balanced translocation	Very rare	2–3%
Translocation G/G 46, XY or XX, —G, +t (GqGq)		Normal	Normal	Most frequent situation 1% for this type	

+t (21/22)	Balanced translocation	Normal	10%
	Normal	Balanced translocation	Small number of observations; 2–4%
+t (21/21)	Balanced translocation	Normal	
	Normal	Balanced translocation	Very rare	100%

---

[a] Data combined from different statistics.

[b] Unless special staining techniques have been used for identification, the laboratory report usually specifies only the group affiliation of the supernumerary chromosome (G)—for example, 46, XY, +G.

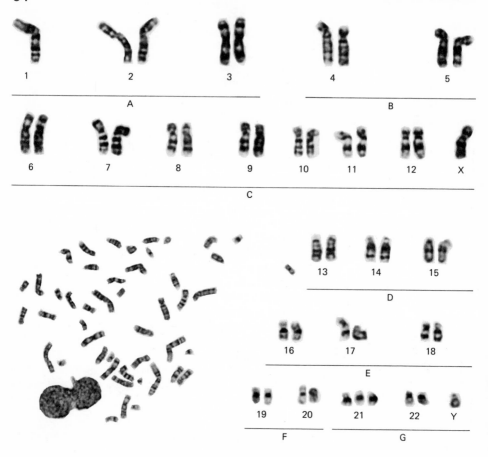

FIGURE 7.2. Photographs of the chromosome complement from a male patient with mongolism. The photograph shows chromosomes at mitosis, specifically, those of metaphase. Division has taken place in all except one location, which is called the centromere area. Whereas the insert photograph on the lower left shows the chromosomes in their natural position, the primary illustration shows them organized according to numbers. One of the chromosomes of the G group is present three times instead of in the normal pair (trisomy). The Y chromosome is also shown. (Modified Giesma stain)

some too many and another having one chromosome too few. Should this gamete be fertilized, the resultant zygote is monosomic and, as a rule, nonviable. On the other hand, if an oocyte with an extra chromosome is fertilized, a trisomy results. A zygote is viable if the triple chromosome is number 21, and it can survive for some time after birth with a trisomy of chromosomes 13 and 18. In general, a trisomy of other chromosomes seems to be lethal except for the sex chromosomes, which are subject to special conditions (see pp. 71–74).

Nondisjunction may occur in the germ cell of either parent. Apparently it occurs more often in the maternal germ cells, and the probability that this will occur increases as the mother gets older. It is therefore not surprising that trisomies of autosomes 13 and 18 as well as those of the sex chromosomes occur more· frequently in older women. Why this should be so is still a mystery.

These facts account for one group of mongoloid children, and we are left with the other group (Fig. 7.1), where the trisomy occurs independently of the age of the mother and where the recurrence frequency is demonstrably higher compared to other women of the same age group.

The first step in explaining these cases was a chromosome analysis. Figure 7.3 shows one of the first pedigrees of this kind. The proband (marked with an arrow in the diagram) had the normal number of chromosomes—46—but one of his D chromosomes (probably number 14) showed elongated short arms. The same peculiarity was noticed in a chromosome analysis of the proband's mongoloid first cousin. The examination of the two normal mothers and the equally normal grandmother solved the mystery. All three women had only 45 chromosomes, but among these was the elongated D chromosome. The missing chromosome was of the G group.

The authors concluded that the elongation of the D chromosome represented the most important parts of the missing chromosome 21. This would result in the women possessing

FIGURE 7.3. Familial occurrence of translocation and mongolism; see text for explanation.

After Carter *et al.* (1960; cited in Vogel, 1961)

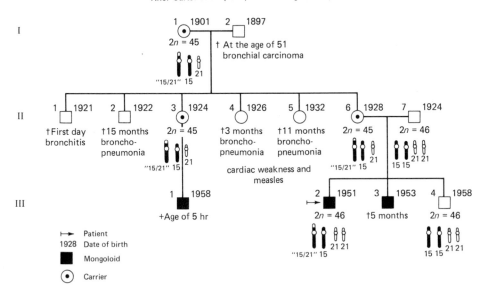

the normal amount of genetic material, whereas the affected children would possess the genetic material three times, similar to patients with a 21-trisomy. Such translocations occur when chromosomes break and the parts rejoin incorrectly (Fig. 7.4).

In practical terms, two types of translocations are important: reciprocal translocations and Robertson's type (centric fusion). In the reciprocal type, chromosome arms of two different chromosomes break off and re-join cross-wise, each with the other chromosome. Thus, the total number of chromosomes remains unchanged, but two of them have a distinctly altered shape. In the Robertsonian type, the centromer regions of acrocentric chromosomes fuse, involving the possible loss of functionally irrelevant chromosome material. Morphologically, the chromosome complement is one short. The above mentioned example of a D/G translocation is of the Robertsonian type. In this case, the chromosome break must have occurred at least three generations ago. A fortunate accident prevented the appearance of mongoloid children in the first two generations despite the fact that the probability was very high. In these cases, the karyotype was balanced. In the third generation, however, the defect manifested itself in three children.

The various behavioral possibilities for such translocation chromosomes during the meiotic divisions are shown in Fig. 7.6. In theory there could be further types of D-chromosome/translocation-chromosome combinations in a germ cell; in fact, they do not seem to occur. An increased miscarriage rate, due to the lethal zygotes, must be expected.

According to the diagram, there is a theoretical 33.3% risk of a mongoloid child if the mother has a balanced karyotype. However, various authors have recently demonstrated with extensive calculations that the actual risk is considerably

1. ROBERTSONIAN TYPE:

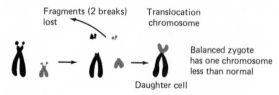

2. RECIPROCAL:

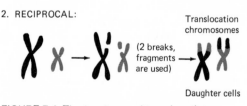

FIGURE 7.4. The two types of translocations.

Karyotype of the
diploid cell

First maturation division

Second maturation
division

Germ cells
(haploid)

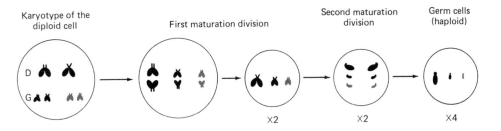

×2   ×2   ×4

FIGURE 7.5. Diagram of the germ cell development in human beings. The diagram shows a pair of D chromosomes (large, black) beside two pairs of G chromosomes (no. 21—small, red; no. 22—small, black). Briefly, meiosis effects are such that each germ cell contains a haploid set of all three chromosomes.

lower. There is also an appreciable difference depending upon which of the parents is the carrier of the balanced karyotype. According to Mikkelsen and Stene (1970), the following risk figures are closer to actuality: for children of female translocation carriers, 10%; for those of male carriers, considerably lower (exact calculations proved impossible). There is also the added risk that the child in turn will have the balanced karyotype. According to these authors, this risk is 57%, regardless of which parent transmits the translocation. Many cases (26 of 59, or almost 50% of the D/G translocation cases in the literature; Mikkelsen, 1971) occur as new mutations. If both parents are free of the translocation, there is no increase of the recurrence risk over and above the figures given in Table 7.1. Recent data reported by Nadler (1972) indicate a slightly higher risk.

Other familial cases with young mothers were later examined; occasionally a D/G translocation was discovered. Apart from this, another form of translocation within the G group itself was observed. The majority of the remaining patients manifested the 21-trisomy.

The development of a G/G translocation can occur in three ways:
1. It may be a 21/22 translocation. This develops in exactly the same manner as shown for the D/G translocation.
2. It may be a 21/21 translocation.
3. The third possibility is a 21 isochromosome.

During meiosis, the situation with a 21/22 translocation is similar to that of D/G translocations. The child-to-be will (a) be phenotypically and genetically normal; (b) be phenotypically normal but the carrier of a balanced translocation; (c) have Down's syndrome.

With the 21/21 translocation and the 21 isochromosome, chances are even worse. The zygote either aborts or it develops into a mongoloid child. There is no possibility that a normal child will be born in such a case (Fig. 7.7).

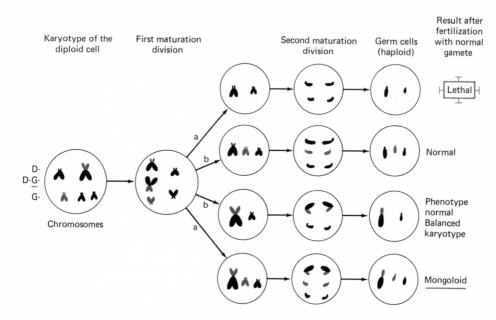

FIGURE 7.6. Diagram of germ cell development when the mother is a D/G translocation carrier—a balanced D/G translocation. One D chromosome shows the translocated long arm of one of the no. 21 chromosomes. Only one single chromosome 21 is present. Since chromosome 21 accidentally combines with the two D chromosomes, four types of germ cells may develop (in descending order): (1) The D chromosome without translocation finds itself in a germ cell which does not have chromosome 21. Lacking this, the fertilized zygote is monosomic and therefore lethal. (2) The D chromosome without translocation finds itself in a germ cell with the normal chromosome 21. This germ cell is normal and results, upon fertilization, in a genotypically and phenotypically normal zygote. (3) The D chromosome with translocation finds itself in a germ cell without chromosome 21. The resultant zygote possesses 45 chromosomes but has a complete (balanced) karyotype. (4) The D chromosome with translocation finds itself in a germ cell with an additional chromosome 21. The resultant zygote therefore possesses 46 chromosomes, but the genetic material for the long arm of chromosome 21 is in a triploid stage and the child will be mongoloid.

By means of the banding-pattern analysis it is possible to differentiate clearly between a 21/22 and a 21/21 transloca-tion. Chromosome 21 shows a strong band of fluorescence on its long arm, whereas chromosome 22 shows only weak fluorescence with maximum intensity located on its short arm and in the centromer region. Using the Giemsa tech-nique, the same bands can be seen as areas of higher density (see Fig. 7.2).

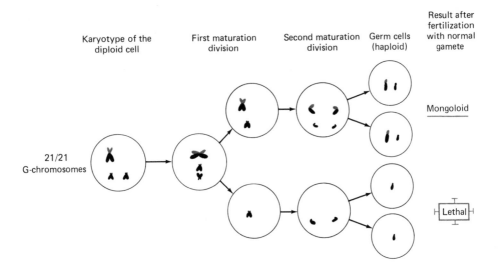

FIGURE 7.7. Formation of germ cells in the case of a 21/21 translocation and 21 isochromosome. In this diagram, one chromosome 21 is red and the other black. Either the translocation or isochromosome finds itself in the germ cell; the resultant zygote has too much genetic material, and the child will be mongoloid. Or the translocation chromosome does not get into the germ cell at all, in which case the zygote has one chromosome too few and is therefore lethal.

On the whole, however, G/G translocations occur spontaneously, i.e., both parents have a normal karyotype. In these cases there is no increase in the risk for future children.

The above observations would lead one to conclude that all patients belonging to the age-independent group are the results of a translocation. That, again, is not the case; these are the figures for the frequency of translocation among the children of young mothers according to Mikkelsen (1971a): Of 1,431 cases of mongolism where the mother's age at birth was below 30, only 115 cases were due to a translocation. Of these, 69 were spontaneous, 32 were hereditary, and in 14 cases the parents could not be examined. Of 1,058 cases where the mother's age at birth was over 30, only 16 were due to translocations: 7 were spontaneous, 5 hereditary, and in 4 cases the parents were not examined. This means that there are women who actually tend to form germ cells with an extra chromosome 21. This may be—and often is—the result of an age-independent tendency toward non-disjunction; but that is not all. There are a few known cases where the mother possesses a cell clone that is trisomic for chromosome 21. If this trisomic cell clone affects only a small fraction of a cells, the mother will appear phenotypically normal; should a part of the ovary be affected, then she may produce a mongoloid child. Individuals with genetically different cell clones in their bodies are called mosaics.

In cases of a mosaic, an accurate genetic prediction is not possible. There is no way of ascertaining how much of the ovary is affected, but this fact alone forces one to assume a greatly increased risk for further defective children.

A relevant detail, at this point, is the fact that cases of mongolism themselves sometimes turn out to be mosaics. When this occurs, it means that the majority of the total body manifest the 21-trisomy. The most important karyotypes involved in mongolism are summarized once more in Fig 7.8. The following conclusions apply to actual counseling:

1. The child is the only member of the family manifesting the anomaly. Its mother was over 35 years of age at the time of birth. In this case, one can assume a 21-trisomy. Chromosome analysis is always indicated if further children are wanted or if siblings are present who may want to know whether they may possibly be carriers. Given easily accessible facilities, the doctor certainly should recommend a chromosome analysis, just to make sure; in this group, translocation carriers, are very rare. The probability of a repetition of the misfortune with future children corresponds to the age-specific risk figures given in Table 7.2. The risk is only slightly increased above the rate for the same age group in the average population.

FIGURE 7.8. The major karyotypes involved in mongolism.

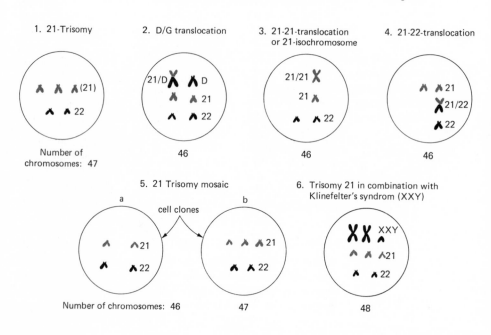

2. The child is the only case within the family but the mother is under 35. In this case, chromosome analysis of the child and its parents is virtually prerequisite. If a translocation manifests itself, its exact nature must be determined and a cytogenetic analysis should be carried out on both parents. For the empiric risk figures, see Table 7.1.

3. There are other cases of mongolism among the siblings or within the closer degrees of kinship; i.e., mongoloid cousins, aunts, uncles, etc. In this case a chromosome analysis of the patient, his parents, and possibly other relatives as well is definitely indicated. Should a translocation be the cause, the above-mentioned criteria apply.

If a 21-trisomy is revealed, despite the mother's normal chromosome complement, and another mongoloid child has already resulted from the same marriage, then one will have to assume a "disposition toward non-disjunction" in one of the parents, presumably the mother. This makes an exact probability prognosis for further children impossible, but the probability is certainly much higher than average.

4. The child is the first case of mongolism in the family but another numerical chromosome anomaly has been found in an earlier child (Klinefelter syndrome; trisomy-13, trisomy-18). In this case, one is again confronted by a "disposition to nondisjunction" with the correspondingly higher probability figures for further sick childen. Several cases of this kind of combination have been recorded.

5. Clinically speaking, the child is mongoloid; cytogenetically, the child is a mosaic. There are no known other cases in the family. As yet, no research results dealing with this specific problem have been published. Until such time, counseling will have to treat such cases as if they were 21- trisomics.

Other Numerical and Structural Chromosome Aberrations

The example of Down's syndrome has served to illustrate the most usual and therefore—practically speaking—most important situations in cases of chromosome aberrations. This part of the chapter will deal with other anomalies that can be traced to morphologically visible chromosome changes. For the sake of clarity and brevity, we will confine ourselves to the most frequent anomalies; detailed discussion of the massed case histories and research data in this area would be out of place in this guide (Hamerton, 1971). However, we would like to point out that in this area, particularly, new discoveries are constantly being made and the consultation of a geneticist in cases of this kind is especially advisable.

ANOMALIES IN SEX DEVELOPMENT

Within this group, anomalies in the sex development of the child are the most frequent, and thus, practically speaking, play the most important role. The first step toward counseling in these cases is to elucidate as far as possible the clinical, endocrinological, and cytogenetic picture of each particular case. The methods of the clinical and endocrinological examinations will not be discussed here; the cytogenetic examination, however, proceeds in two stages: (1) The determination of the sex chromatin. (2) If no clear diagnosis results, then chromosome analysis, despite the time and cost involved, must be done.

Determination of the sex chromatin is usually done by examing the epithelial cells of the oral mucosa or of the hair-sheath, and by counting the drumsticks on the granulocytes. Individuals with two (or more) X chromosomes (i.e., normally women) have the so-called Barr body or sex chromatin in the majority of their body cells. They are chromatin-positive. Some, a small percentage, of the granulocytes show drumstick-shaped appendages; hence the term "drumstick."

Normal males do not have these chromatin bodies since they possess only one X chromosome. In male cells, on the other hand, the heterochromatic part of the Y chromosome can be recognized from its strong fluorescence after dyeing with fluorescent stains (Y bodies). Thus, it is possible to determine the sex of an individual through the morphological analysis of the cell nucleus—at least insofar as the examined cells are concerned. This latter qualification is necessary since human beings do not necessarily have the same genetic sex in all their cells. They might be mosaics for different cell clones.

Although the test methods for Barr bodies and drumsticks are relatively simple, a great deal of experience is required in order to reduce the likelihood of error. As a rule, it is advisable to employ a laboratory specializing in such tests.

Chromosome analysis allows us to class sex-development anomalies in one of two major categories: those with and those without aberrations in the number or structure of chromosomes. In a practical case, the ascertainment of these facts allows us to derive the following rule of thumb: *If a child manifests more or less than the normal number of sex chromosomes and the parents are genetically normal, then the probability of a recurrence of the phenomenon in future children is unchanged or only negligibly higher than that of the average population. If the patient's number of chromosomes is normal, then the risk for future children may be greater—but not necessarily so—as other genetic conditions may be involved.* For the patients themselves, counseling is usually redundant: as a rule, they are sterile. We will now discuss some of the more frequent anomalies individually.

Klinefelter's syndrome is characterized by 47 chromosomes and the karyotype XXY. A few cases resembling Klinefelter's syndrome have even more X chromosomes. This means that the epithelial cells possess Barr bodies and leucocytes have drumsticks. As in the 21-trisomy in mongolism, the increased number of X chromosomes is usually the result of non-disjunction during meiosis. Logically, therefore, the frequency of occurrence of this anomaly increases with the age of the mother.

A familial massing of non-disjunction resulting in Klinefelter's syndrome has not as yet been established with any degree of certainty. Therefore, the birth of such a child does not mean that the answer to the question of further children must be negative. In fact, such advice would usually come far too late anyway, since the condition is usually not evident and consequently undiagnosed during the early years of the patient's life.

Despite this, one must always keep in mind that there have been families with various cases of different trisomies, and that there are patients who suffer from mongolism as well as Klinefelter's syndrome. These observations support the theory that there are genetic factors which constitute a non-disjunction disposition. This results in a comparatively pessimistic genetic prognosis for a woman who has given birth to two children with different trisomies, or who has close relatives (mother, sister) who also have children suffering from trisomies. However, no exact figures as to the probability are available. Therefore, the presence of a child with Klinefelter's syndrome also belongs to the indications for a prenatal diagnosis.

Rarer than the chromatin-positive "real" Klinefelter's syndrome are the cases with tubular fibrosis of the testes, also called the "false" Klinefelter's syndrome. These patients' chromatin tests show negative results, and they have the normal number of chromosomes. A biopsy of the testes will also show the difference between this disease and the "real" Klinefelter's syndrome. This condition, however, has been observed to recur within the same family and among brothers. The probability of further sons with this condition is therefore considerably higher than further cases of the real Klinefelter's syndrome, even though the specific mode of inheritance has not been established and empiric risk figures are unavailable.

In the majority of cases of Klinefelter's syndrome, the chromosome tests give idential results, but this is not the case with the corresponding group of diseases affecting the female sex, the gonadal dysgeneses. Of course, the diagnosis is helped by the fact that the phenotypical sex and the sex-chromatin test results do not concur. In these cases, the apparent sex is female, wheras the Barr bodies and the drumsticks are missing.

Nonetheless, karyotyping does not always lead to the clear confirmation of an XO karyotype. These cases have only 45 chromosomes in all their tissues; they have an X chromosome but lack the Y. Unfortunately, a very strong minority manifests itself as mosaic for two or more cell clones; i.e., XO and XX, XO/XY. XO/XXX, and many more. Mosaics of this sort are more frequent with the gonadal dysgeneses than with Klinefelter's syndrome.

This difference can probably be traced to the different origins of the aberrations. The XO type is usually the result of nondisjunction in the newly fertilized zygote; i.e., during very early cleavage instead of during meiosis. This also explains why this disease is independent of the mother's age.

In comparison with the frequency of sporadic cases of Turner's syndrome, there are hardly any records of familial incidence in cases with chromosome aberrations. However, a single case of this disease within a family is an indication to recommend a prenatal diagnosis. But, just as with Klinefelter's syndrome, the prognosis will be far more pessimistic should there be more than one case in the family, or should other numerical chromosome aberrations have occurred.

It is necessary to distinguish cases of chromosomally caused Turner's syndrome from (admittedly rare) cases of simple gonadal dysgenesis with chromatin-positive nuclei and normal body size. These cases manifest a normal female karyotype XX, but the recurrence of this disease among sisters has been repeatedly recorded. Despite the fact that the mode of inheritance remain uncertain, statistics indicate the necessity for caution in counseling families with this problem.

A further numerical sex chromosome anomaly is the XYY type. Such men are remarkable for their sheer physical size. The anomaly occurs with increased frequency among persons who tend to get into trouble with the law. Sons, however, have so far only been observed to inherit a single Y chromosome and are therefore normal.

The number of anomalies in sex development without a consistent chromosome aberration pattern are legion. The only advice for the general practitioner is "Consult a specialist." There are so many forms, many of which do have genetic roots, that specialized knowledge is required for family counseling.

For cases of an anomaly in sex development, especially those cases that show a normal number of chromosomes, an examination of an entire family is a prerequisite to any counseling. But, and this is a very important but, *negative results from a family examination do not prove that the anomaly in question does not have a genetic cause; it does not mean that the prognosis will necessarily be favorable.*

OTHER AUTOSOMAL ABERRATIONS

We have already discussed the autosomal chromosome aberrations involved in mongolism in great detail. Apart from mongolism, there are only three other clinically important and well-defined autosomal trisomy syndromes: the D-chromosome trisomy (Patau's syndrome), the chromosome-18 trisomy (Edward's syndrome) and trisomy 8. These trisomies lead to such severe and multiple malformations that affected children almost invariably die, at the very latest sometime during infancy. Consequently, there are no offspring. If a mother gives birth to such a child, as far as we know, there is no reason to advise against further children. The same applies to a miscarriage or a stillbirth where a chromosome anomaly is the major cause. The only reservation that must be remembered is the case of a family in which more than one trisomy has occurred. If that happens, then the prognosis for future children will be much less favorable.

Besides the example of numerical autosomal aberrations, there is a large collection of data about various structural aberrations. Many translocations could be traced back for several generations. As long as a corresponding deletion on another chromosome leads to a balanced karyotype, these translocations do not become manifest. It is only when the random division of chromosomes during meiosis creates an unbalanced karyotype that the anomaly appears. Contrary to the Robertsonian type, these translocations are usually of the reciprocal variety (Fig. 7.4).

Carriers with a balanced karyotype have the normal number of chromosomes. Patients with an unbalanced karyotype are usually affected to such a degree that the question of procreation does not arise. The risk figures for children of balanced carriers can be derived from the data in Table 7.2. The data represent an evaluation by Ford and Clegg (1969) of all cases reported in the literature up to 1967. Their calculations seem to disregard the proband selection factor. Their risk figures for phenotypically abnormal children and balanced translocation carriers are therefore probably slightly higher than the actual risk. All the same, the risk for children of balanced translocation carriers is very high indeed, and counseling in such cases will involve making this very clear. However, prenatal diagnosis could provide a way for such a couple to have a healthy child.

Centric fusions of the type D/D, especially those between chromosomes 13 and 14, are still more frequent. The balanced state does not impair the carriers in any recognizable way. During germ cell formation, however, germ cells with the following karyotypes can be formed.

1. Normal karyotype
2. Balanced 13/14 translocation (carrier)
3. Monosomy 13
4. Monosomy 14
5. Translocation trisomy 14
6. Translocation trisomy 13

Of these, (1) and (2) are clinically normal; (3), (4), and (5)

Table 7.2 Outcome of 561 Pregnancies in Matings of Presumptive Translocation Heterozygous Parents[a]

Sex of heterozygous parent	Number of cases	Live birth: normal phenotype			Stillbirth or live birth with abnormal phenotype	Spontaneous abortion
		Translocation heterozygous	Normal karyotype	Chromosomes not investigated		
Male	55	53 (37.9%)[b]	30 (21.4%)[b]	7 (5.0%)[b]	50 (35.7%)[b]	33
Female	106	79 (26.4%)	56 (18.7%)	43 (14.4%)	121 (40.5%)	89
Total	161	132 (30.1%)	86 (19.6%)	50 (11.4%)	171 (39.0%)	122

[a]Data from Ford and Clegg (1969).
[b]Percentages added, with exception of spontaneous abortions.

lead to spontaneous abortion; (6) corresponds clinically to trisomy-13 (D-trisomy). Miscarriage is also frequent, but some children survive up to early infancy. According to Dutrillaux and Lejeune (1970), 25% of pregnancies with D/D translocation end in miscarriages; 2% of children born alive show trisomy-13; trisomy-21 (Down's syndrome) was seen in 2% ("disturbed chromosome balance"). Among the clinically normal children, normal and balanced karyotypes were observed with equal frequencies.

There remain those malformations caused by chromosome deletion; in other words, a piece of chromosome is simply missing. The best-known syndrome of this category is the Cri-du-chat (Cat cry) syndrome, named after the characteristic high monotonous cry of the affected infant. This disease is caused by a deletion of the short arm of chromosome 5. Patients, apart from other symptoms, are also mentally deficient. An increased recurrence risk in the same sibship exists only in families with translocations.

Spontaneous and Recurrent Abortions

According to common estimates, 15 to 25% of all pregnancies terminate in recognizable spontaneous abortions. Of these, an unknown but sizable proportion are caused by genetic disorders. When a miscarriage occurs, the first step will always be a gynecological evaluation followed by therapy if the cause can be ascribed to a functional or morphological anomaly of the genital tract. Even if no overt cause can be found, an isolated miscarriage is not usually a matter of grave concern. However, if the event recurs, the causes should be investigated more thoroughly.

A certain percentage of natural abortions is caused by genetic lethals. Examples of such lethals are autosomal-dominant new mutations, X-chromosomal mutations (or lethal hemizygotes with dominant X-chromosomal defects), and autosomal-recessive homozygotes. Unless the responsible anomaly can be diagnosed in the fetus itself, the diagnosis must be based on evidence derived from the pedigree. Part of the increased abortion rate in consanguineous marriages, for instance, will be due to homozygosity of autosomal-recessive lethals.

Between 20 and 37% of all recognizable spontaneous abortions, particularly those of the first trimester, are caused by chromosomal anomalies (Carr, 1969; Larson and Titus, 1970; Pawlowitzki, 1972). In general, these represent de novo events arising in some stage of meiosis or errors in early mitotic divisions. A genetic predisposition for such events has been found in a few families, but on the whole, such de novo events will not indicate a higher than average risk for subsequent pregnancies. It is well established that phenotypically normal persons are sometimes the carriers of balanced chromosomal anomalies. Such a condition will result in the forma-

tion of unbalanced germ cells in gametogenesis in a calculable proportion of all the gametes formed. The unbalanced
karyotype will either prove lethal and abort, or it will result in
a defective child. This is unquestionably so for translocations
of the DqGq type. There is conflicting evidence in regard to
t(DqDq) translocations in that Court-Brown (1967), evaluating
a limited number of families, found a 35% abortion rate for
the progeny of male carriers and a 43% one for those of female carriers. Hamerton (1968), on the other hand, found no
increase in the spontaneous abortion rate for families of carriers with a balanced Robertsonian translocation. This discrepancy may be partly due to a bias in the case collection;
more probably, it can be ascribed to the fact that the individual D chromosomes involved have not been indentified in
the examined families. In any case, it is to be expected that
chromosome aberrations will be more frequent when the
recurrent miscarriages are not due to gynecological or other
physical abnormalities. This explanation is particularly probable if the pedigree shows at least one abnormal offspring
apart from the recurrent abortions.

From the limited number of published studies, it seems
reasonable to assume that 2 to 4% of recurrent abortions are
due to an unbalanced karyotype of a parent. Therefore, if a
woman has two or more abortions, the karyotype of the
aborted conceptus should be determined. If an anomaly is
found or the karyotype cannot be established, both parents
should have their chromosomes analyzed. A parent's chromosomal translocation or inversion may be responsible for the
recurrent abortions. Inversions can be recognized only if they
are searched for very carefully. Special techniques (banding,
fluorescent staining) may be required. An exact diagnosis is
important because the risk involved concerns not only the
recurrence of abortions, but also the possible birth of malformed and defective children. No general risk figures can be
given since there are very few data. Each case must be analyzed separately (Bhasin et al., 1973).

Appendix   The nomenclature for description of human karyotypes has
been regulated by international agreement. First, the total
number of chromosomes is given, followed by the sex chromosome complement. Then, which chromosomes are too
many, or too few, or structurally altered is indicated. Some
examples:

46, XX	Normal female karyotype;
46, XY	Normal male karyotype;
47, +G	Male karyotype with 47 chromosomes; one G chromosome too many.
47, XY, +21	As above; the additional chromosome has been identified as 21.

46, XY, 1q+	Male karyotype with 46 chromosomes; the long arm (q) of one chromosome 1 is larger than normal.
46, XX, 5p−	Female karyotype with 46 chromosomes; the short arm (p) of one chromosome 5 is shorter than normal.
45, X	Karyotype with 45 chromosomes only; only one X chromosome present.
45, XX, −D, −G, +t (DqGq)	Female karyotype with 45 chromosomes; one typical D and one typical G are lacking; instead, there is a chromosome that consists of the long arms of one D and one G chromosome (balanced Robertsonian translocation between the long arms of one Y and one G).

8 Malformations Not Subject to a Simple Mode of Inheritance

The birth of a malformed child is the most common reason for consulting a doctor as to the chances of further children manifesting the same defect. In most cases, the answer is simply that the occurrence is accidental and a repetition in the family is as unlikely as lightning striking twice in the same place. This answer satisfies the doctor's responsibility to reassure the frequently deeply disturbed parents—and it may even be the correct answer. But, as with lightning, some houses are, for very definite reasons, more endangered than others, and it is the business of the doctor to eliminate the possibility of such reasons or to evaluate them correctly where they do exist. Reassurance on any other grounds would be negligent, not to say irresponsible.

The first thing to be clarified is the question of whether the malformation belongs to a particular syndrome or category of defects with a simple mode of inheritance. Some examples have been given: achondroplasia (p. 28), Marfan's syndrome (p. 28), Apert's syndrome (acrocephalosyndactyly; p. 29). This will require the consultation of the relevant literature on the subject. A further step would be to eliminate the possibility of a chromosome aberration (see Chapter 7). The first indication that this suspicion is correct means that the requisite series of specialized tests must be made. Blood or tissue can be sent to distant laboratories. Even tissue taken from the umbilical cord, the amnion, or the fresh corpse can be used for this purpose.

The particular conditions for the transport of such specimens are best discussed with the laboratory that is to carry out the tests. It is generally advisable to check back with the laboratory in any case, since such tests are very complicated and laboratory capacity is limited. The trouble is that these samples must be processed immediately. Specialized laboratories of this kind can usually be found in the genetics departments of larger universities, some children's hospitals, gynecological clinics, and university departments of anatomy and/or pathology. Table 8.1 contains general indications for chromosome analysis.

After all these possibilities have been exhausted, it is very possible that none of them will have provided a satisfactory explanation. A great number of malformations belong in none of the above named categories. The first question in such a case is, could the malformation possibly have an exogenous cause? Rubella embryopathy as the consequence of a virus disease (German measles) and the thalidomide embryopathy as a drug-induced malformation are cases in point for purely exogenous disturbances in embryonic development; but such textbook cases are rare. There are very few other exogenous agents that can be blamed with as much certainty. Before one can even consider an exogenous cause for a defect, one has to make sure that the suggested event occurred at a time during embryonic development when the particular malformation in question could still take place. After all, the development of the specific organ might already have been completed (Fig. 8.1).

Even recurring malformations can sometimes be traced to permanently present exogenous factors within the mother, such as a repeatedly disturbed implantation of the egg in the uterus. For toxoplasmosis, teratogenic effects of a latent infection have been suggested.

The type of malformation that results depends decisively, too, on the time at which the supposed exogenous event took place. It is therefore very unlikely that the same or very similar malformations among siblings can be explained through exogenous factors alone.

Table 8.1

Common stigmata of autosomal chromosome anomalies
  1. Low birth weight (small for date)
  2. Mental and physical retardation
  3. Multiple malformations (including congenital disease)
  4. Dysplasia of ears, hands
  5. Facial peculiarities (funny-looking child)
  6. Dermatoglyphic anomalies

Symptoms not caused by anomaly of autosomes
  1. Mental retardation without additional malformations
  2. Malformations or dysplasia associated with
     normal mental capacity
  3. Isolated single malformations

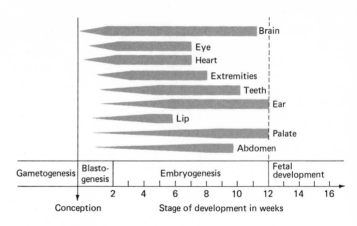

FIGURE 8.1. The relative duration of development of the various human organs during embryogenesis.

After Krone (1961); for more exact and detailed data, see the table by Pliess (cited in Fuhrmann, 1965)

In every retrospective case history of a pregnancy, the re-called "problems and shocks" must be taken with a grain of salt. All too commonly and too often do mother and doctor reassure themselves by blaming some banal and totally ir-relevant occurrence during the pregnancy for the malforma-tion. Apart from that, it is also possible that an exogenous factor merely acted as a catalyst in the sense that the dis-turbance of the pregnancy allowed a genetically determined weakness to manifest itself in an actual malformation. In cases of this sort it is essential not to oversimplify and not to be trapped by the simple either/or formula of *either* exogenous *or* genetic.

The development of the human embryo requires such precise coordination of so many factors and such exact timing of the various processes that it is only too comprehensible that even minute deviations at various points can, at the worst, sum total into a disturbance which cannot be compen-sated—a malformation.

These theoretical concepts were extensively sustained by C. O. Carter's research into congenital pyloric hypertrophy and stenosis. He managed to establish that this disease, which used to be fatal to many infants (before Ramsted's operation), was caused by a so-called multifactorial system, the com-bined activity of numerous genes. (The same applies to a number of other congenital malformations, such as the con-genital dislocation of the hip, which was mentioned earlier.)

In our discussion of simple modes of inheritance, it was possible to consider the responsible gene in isolation. The dis-cussion made the sweeping basic assumption that a particular

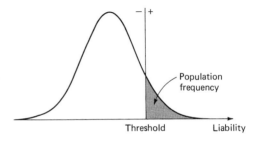

FIGURE 8.2

Principle of the multifactorial mode of inheritance with threshold effect: the continuously (in our example, normal) distributed liability results in a manifestation of a pathological phenotype as soon as a "threshold" has been passed.

gene alone is responsible for a particular trait and that other genes at other gene loci do not affect its expressivity at all. Strictly speaking, this is hardly ever entirely correct. When the expressivity of a trait is dependent upon other genes, even if only to a very limited extent, one speaks of major and minor genes.

For genetic traits outside the simple modes of inheritance, it is frequently true that their manifestation is dependent upon a number of genes, each of which contributes relatively little to the total variation. What is even more confusing, the contribution of each gene is nonspecific; only the total effect is finally visible. This type of causality is called additive polygeny or, more generally, the multifactorial mode of inheritance. Each individual gene remains within the Mendelian framework as discussed in relation to the simple modes of inheritance. Therefore, the more numerous the genes involved in the expression of a trait, the more in evidence will be a continuous gradation in the variation of trait expressivity. The trait distribution is thus unimodal in the manner of a normal distribution.

In other cases, a trait only manifests itself after an unspecified number of genes have been involved—and then only conditionally. Especially in the case of a malformation, such "tolerance limits" are easily imaginable; we call them threshold values. The phenotype is alternately distributed (normal–abnormal), whereas the underlying genetic liability shows a quantitatively continuous gradation in its variation. Among

FIGURE 8.3

The share of common genes possessed by close relatives of a proband, by reason of their common ancestry.

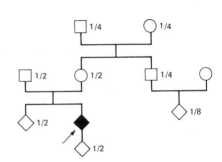

relatives, the degree of liability would correspond to the number of commonly inherited genes.

Carter's research was based on the fact that congenital pyloric stenosis is much more common with male than with female infants. At the same time, the total evidence showed that pyloric stenosis appeared with far greater frequency among the close relatives of affected girls than among the corresponding relatives of affected boys. Neither exogenous factors nor any simple mode of inheritance could account for this peculiarity. The pattern, however, becomes perfectly logical as soon as one postulates a quantitative distribution of the genetic liability for pyloric stenosis, i.e., the involvement of a large number of genes. If, as it seems, unspecific sex-dependent factors inhibit the manifestation of the anomaly in girls, then it follows that affected girls are subject to a particularly strong genetic liability, i.e., that they possess many of the responsible genes. Since half the genes are common among first degree relatives, those of affected girls will possess more of the responsible genes than those of affected boys (Table 8.2).

For practical counseling in cases of malfunctions outside the simple modes of inheritance, we are forced to resort to empiric risk figures. These figures are based on the statistical data gained from research into sufficiently large random series of the relatives of patients with a particular anomaly. Theoretically, one could object that such series simply do not permit the elimination of familial nongenetic factors, but then genetic counseling is primarily concerned with establishing the repetition probability of an anomaly. *Much more serious and valid is the objection that the risk is specific for every family and therefore varies from case to case. The series could thus include a number of families with a very high specific risk together with a greater number of families with a much smaller specific risk.* This would result in comparatively low risk figures that would prove inaccurate in all cases, since the

Table 8.2 Pyloric Stenosis: Frequency among the Close Relatives of Male and Female Probands

Number and sex of the probands	Brother	Sister	Son	Daughter	Nephew	Niece	Cousin male	Cousin female
♂ 281	5/230 2.17%	5/242 2.07%	19/296 6.42%	7/274 2.55%	5/231 2.16%	1/213 0.47%	6/1061 0.57%	3/1043 0.29%
♀ 149	11/101 10.89%	9/101 8.91%	14/61 22.95%	7/62 11.48%	4/60 6.67%	1/78 1.28%	6/745 0.81%	2/694 0.29%

Data, somewhat abbreviated, from Carter (1964).

calculations are based on an assumption of risk equality for all the families. There is also no way of determining whether the proband's family belongs to the especially endangered group or not, unless further malformations of the same or a related nature in other members of the family indicate it. As a general rule, the risk for the recurrence of a defect in the relatives, in a situation where the multifactorial mode of inheritance seems to apply, is to some degree related to the severity of manifestation in the index case.

Remaining uncertainties can only be removed gradually, as larger series are carefully examined and criteria for subgroups are established. However, when one is confronted with the necessity of making a decision, the statistics for malformations from series so far available will at least give an approximation. Table 8.3 is only a representative selection of some of the more thoroughly examined anomalies to date. *Counseling in any particular case will require the consultation of the most recent literature on the subject.* Some of the older series contain considerable errors in the mode of ascertainment and the statistical evaluation of the data.

Let it be said here and now that there are no "common" or "average" probability figures with these malformations. A general estimate—but it is only an approximation—would place the risk of the recurrence of an anomaly in a family where there are no other cases and the parents are normal at 3 to 5%. Should there already be two children with the same defect, then the risk increases to a value somewhere between 5 and 25%, and in several diseases has been found to be about 10%.

In order not to overestimate these figures, one should always remember that all children, including those of "perfectly normal" families, run an approximately 1 to 2% risk of being born with a serious malformation. Even here, it is impossible to give exact figures, since there is neither a commonly accepted definition of what constitutes a "serious malformation" nor common criteria for ascertainment and diagnosis. Simply adding the frequencies of the different malformations taken separately does not help either, since this method would leave out multiple malformations. Besides, the figures include the children from families with a definitely established genetic liability.

For counseling purposes there is no point in trying to calculate risk figures to the fraction of a percentage, however desirable this may be in research. It is the major task of the counselor to find the closest applicable average figure and to make sure that the case in question does not belong to those defect groups with a particularly high risk or even simple Mendelian inheritance. Clinical features in the family history may help to clarify the category to which the defect belongs.

Table 8.3 Empiric Risk for Common Malformations Not Showing Simple Mendelian Inheritance

Type of malformation	Incidence among live born (%)	Incidences of same or related malformation (%)			References
		Siblings	Children	First cousins	
Anencephaly[a]		5.0% for anence-phaly and spina bifida			Penrose (1957)
	~0.14%				Carter and Evans (1971)
Spina bifida	~0.1	5.1			Hindse-Nielsen (1938); Carter and Evans (1971)
	~0.16				
Anencephaly, spina bifida and/or hydrocephaly, combined[b]	~0.29	1.89 (including 4.9 stillborn and prema-ture)			Record and McKeown (1960) Degenhardt (1964)
	~0.3	4.7			Carter and Evans (1971)
If one child is affected after birth of two affected children		4.0			Carter and Roberts (1967)
		10.0			
Isolated cleft palate[a]	~0.02–0.05	1.8–2.3 (higher for siblings of males)	7.0%	0.2%	Fraser (1955, 1970)
If parent is affected also		17.0			Schulze (1964)
Harelip and cleft palate (cheilognathopalatoschisis)	~0.1–0.18 ♂ > ♀				Fogh-Andersen (1942, 1964); Fraser (1970); Hanhart and Kælin (1972)
If one child is affected		3.5–4.4 (~8.0) (higher for siblings of females)	2.0–3.5		

Defect	Frequency (%)	Risk for sibs (%)	Risk for offspring (%)
If parent is affected also			14.0
After birth of two affected children			9.0
(In general, risk increases with severity of defect in proband)			
Congenital heart diseases in general (if not part of syndrome or special type with better known transmission)	~0.8	2–5	2–4
After birth of two affected children		5.5–8.0	
Vetr. Sept. Def.	~0.2	1–2 (?)	1–4
Atrial Sept. Def. (special types excluded; autosomal-dominant in some families)			1–4
Fallot's tetralogy	~0.031	1–4	
Pulm. stenosis	~0.06	1–3	
Pat. duct. art.	~0.08	2–4 (PDA 2.3)	2–4 (PDA 2.5)
Transposition of great vessels	~0.08	4–5 for CHD in general; 1–2 for TGV	
Tricuspid atresia	~0.02	~1.0 (?)	
Valv. aortic stenosis (subvalv. and supravalv. stenosis excluded)	~0.02–0.04	2–4	
Coarctation of aorta	0.02–0.04	1–3	1–3

Reviews: Fuhrmann (1972a, b); Jörgensen (1972); Zetterqvist (1972)

Table 8.3 Empiric Risk for Common Malformations Not Showing Simple Mendelian Inheritance (continued)

Type of malformation	Incidence among live born (%)	Incidences of same or related malformation (%)			References
		Siblings	Children	First cousins	
Pyloric stenosis	See Table 8.2				
Congenital intestinal aganglionosis ("M. Hirschsprung") (for more exact figures the length of the aganglionic segment should be considered, see ref.)	0.02 ♂ > ♀	0.6–18 of ♂♂ 6.3; 2.0 ♂ ♀ of ♀♀ 10.4; 4.4			Passarge (1972)
Hypospadias	♂ 0.1 to 0.3	brothers, 9.6 9.5–10.5		0.7	Sorensen (1953); Lenz (1964); Chen and Wooley, Jr. (1971)
Congenital dislocation of the hip	0.3	♂ ♀ 1 11 (in general, higher in higher social classes)	♂ ♀ 6 17	0.3	Wynne-Davies (1970) [See Table 1.2 for data of Carter (1964), somewhat at variance]
If one child and one parent is affected		36			
Clubfoot	0.1	2.9–3.1 of ♀♀ 5.97 of ♂♂ 1.95		0.2	Idelberger (1939); Grebe (1964); Wynne-Davies (1964); Carter (1965)

[a]Single families with apparently monogenic inheritance have been reported.
[b]In boys with hydrocephalus, the X-chromosomal recessive type must be excluded.

Important examples are the rare cases of X-linked recessive hydrocephalus in boys with aqueductal stenosis, usually not associated with spina bifida, but frequently showing a flection deformity of the thumb; or the occasional family with an autosomal-recessive inheritance of anencephaly and myelomeningocele, as reported by Fuhrmann *et al* (1971). Other examples are the not infrequent families with an apparently dominant inheritance of the atrial septal defect, sometimes associated with upper limb deformity (Oram-Holt syndrome), or the dominant sex-limited inheritance of hypospadias in the hypertelorism-hyperspadias syndrome (Opitz syndrome).

Example 7: Normal, unrelated parents had as their first child a son with a grave congenital malformation of the heart. A cardiological examination showed a ventricular septal defect and a pseudotruncus aortalis; i.e., Fallot's tetralogy combined with pulmonary atresia. Four years later a girl was born and died soon after birth. A postmortem showed another grave—this time fatal—malformation of the heart, Eisenmenger's complex. There were no other known cases of malformation in the immediate family or within the further removed degree of kinship. At this point, the sterilization of the wife was being considered. The decisive questions are as follows:

1. What are the chances that further children from this marriage will manifest the same or a similar malformation?
2. Are the chances such that further children should not be conceived?
3. Is sterilization either indicated or justified?

Let us consider question 1: It is certain that genetic factors are extensively involved in cases of congenital heart disease. A few types with a simple mode of inheritance are known, but these specific malformations are outside this category. For most of the cardiac defects, the causes are infinitely complex. We are therefore obliged to rely on the available empiric risk figures. Until recently, the only figures available applied to families with one affected child (see Table 8.3). As the table shows, even here the results are not entirely in agreement. The reason for this may be different modes of ascertainment, but perhaps it is simply a matter of the accidental selection of patients constituting the series. Moreover, some of the series were very small. A mean assumption figure would rate the recurrence risk at 2.5%.

However, within the group of congenital heart diseases there are apparently definite differences. For the particular combination found in our family there are no specific data, but it is obvious that the various components of these malformations correspond to those specific defects which manifest a higher risk. Had we been asked about the probability figures after birth of the first child, the answer would have been that the chances lay somewhere between 2 to 3.5–4%.

Meanwhile, a second child has manifested a similar malformation. This proves that for this family, genetic factors are decisive and not merely subordinate and partial components. Just the same, to postulate a simple mode of inheritance would be to jump to conclusions. A possibility in this direction would be the autosomal-recessive mode of inheritance with a resultant 25% risk for further children (see p. 37). Another possibility—somewhat more remote—would be an autosomal-dominant mode of inheritance with *extremely* weak penetrance, with a resultant relative risk of considerably less than 1/2, probably less than 1/4. These two alternatives, however, represent the worst possible extent of the risk involved. Asked about the average probability of recurrence, we should base ourselves only on series giving the empiric risk figures compiled on the basis of families with two affected children.

To date, two such series, evaluating cases in 21 and 54 families, respectively, are available. According to these series, the calculated risk is somewhere between 5 and 10%, depending upon one's assumptions in relation to the ascertainment modalities used. A risk of 5 to 8% would be a justifiable prognosis in this particular case (see Table 8.3). At the same time one would have to mention the potentially higher risk for some families.

The second question, given these facts, has no clear answer and should not be answered without knowledge and discussion of the very particular situation and the personalities involved. Personal considerations would probably be the deciding factors.

Should the couple decide against further children, the third question would have to be answered: Is a surgical sterilization indicated? Again, the particular family situation would have to be considered; but in nearly all cases, normal contraceptive methods will suffice. The steroid ovulation inhibitors, if employed conscientiously, are virtually as effective as sterilization. Only where the patient's constitution, for some reason, cannot tolerate the steroid contraceptives despite professional prescription and a long period of trial, and there are serious objections to other conservative contraceptive methods, should sterilization be considered at all. Another important consideration would be the age of the particular couple, for the situation might arise that children are ardently desired in a second marriage. Sterilization is nearly always irreversible.

9 Prenatal Diagnosis

At this point, it seems appropriate to sketch briefly the possibilities and limitations of tests for the prenatal diagnosis of genetic defects. This field of research has been expanding rapidly in recent years. We will not discuss the highly technical details here but will confine ourselves to the facts that a practicing physician should know. The tests and the diagnosis itself will, in any case, be carried out by specialized laboratories [for methodological details, see Emery (1970); Dorfman (1972); *Birth Defects*, Orig. Art. Ser. Vol. VII, (1971).]

The most common and most successful test method for prenatal diagnosis is the examination of amnion cells. Amniotic fluid is extracted by way of a suprapubic amniocentesis (the penetration of the amnion sac above the symphysis with a hollow needle). The process is almost painless. The timing of such a test is usually a practical compromise: the earlier a successful test is made, the earlier the condition of the embryo will be known; the later it is left, the more likely it is that sufficient amnion cells for a successful test will be found. Unfortunately, the culturing of the cells takes time, sometimes up to a few weeks. Emery (1970) suggests somewhere between the 12th and the 20th week of pregnancy as the best time. Most authors are agreed on the period between the 14th and the 16th week. There is some disagreement as to the amount of fluid to be extracted—between 5 and 20 ml—but this is only to be expected, since the total amount of amniotic fluid available depends upon the stage of the pregnancy. At 12 weeks, for instance, there are only about 50 ml of fluid in the amnion sac. The test involves no danger for the prospective mother; the risk of inducing a miscarriage seems to be less than 1%. The amnion fluid is centrifuged and the extracted cells are cultured. The diagnosis is possible only if these cells multiply in sufficient quantity, and thus culturing takes some time, often a few weeks. Research is now in progress to try to find a way to shorten this time.

The indications for a prenatal diagnosis are (1) a high risk of a numerical or structural chromosome anomaly; (2) the increased probability for one of the enzyme defects that can be detected in amnion cells. Since there is an almost 1% chance of injury to the fetus through the amniocentesis, such tests are indicated only if the specific genetic risk is clearly above 1%. Among such cases are chromosome anomalies if (a) one of the parents is the carrier of a balanced translocation; (b) there is already one child with a trisomy syndrome by the same parents; (c) one of the parents is mosaic for a numerical chromosome anomaly; or (d) the prospective mother is older than 38. Also, defects with simple Mendelian inheritance if (a) a former child suffers from an autosomal-recessive metabolic defect that can be diagnosed in amnion cells (see Table 9.1); (b) both parents are, after special examination (see Table 5.1), considered at least probable heterozygotes for such a recessive anomaly; (c) the pedigree provides other evidence indicating a high risk for the child (this may be, but must not be the case, if there is parental consanguinity or origin from a region with extensive inbreeding), or (d) the potential defect is a sex-linked recessive anomaly. As a rule, only male children are affected, and though the tests do not as yet allow us to diagnose the specific defect, the sex of the embryo can be established. In cases where there is already one son with such a defect and independent tests or the pedigree show that the mother is probably (tests) or certainly (daughter of a patient) heterozygous, the determination of the sex of the fetus would simplify the decision of whether to interrupt the pregnancy or not.

Apart from testing for chromosome anomalies and biochemical defects in amnion cells, methods are being developed that will allow us to determine the condition of the embryo from the constitution of the amniotic fluid. Here, determination of the α_1-fetoprotein has become especially useful during recent years. In most cases, we are now able to diagnose anencephaly and/or spina bifida early enough for artificial pregnancy termination. In these conditions, α_1-fetoprotein, which is usually present in small traces, shows such a massive increase that the diagnosis can be made only a few hours after amnioncentesis. The examination is being carried out in an increasing number of laboratories. However, there is one limitation: completely closed defects (about 10% of all cases) cannot be recognized with this method; it requires an open connection between the body of the fetus and the amniotic fluid. Therefore, it is not possible to promise families complete elimination of the risk. It is possible, on the other hand, to explain to them that children with milder conditions will go unrecognized, and they can in most cases be treated successfully. The doctor should therefore explain this possibility to every couple who have already had a child with spina bifida and/or anencephaly.

It is also already possible to obtain information about the shape and movements of the embryo by examining the uterus with ultrasonic waves. This method already permits us to diagnose specific malformations like anencephaly. There are already several cases on record where anencephaly was suc-

Table 9.1 Genetic Diseases for Which Prenatal Diagnosis Has Already Been Successfully Carried Out (*), and Those for Which Present Methods Should Also Prove Adequate

Disorders of lipid metabolism
Fabry disease*
Gaucher disease*
G^{m1} Gangliosidosis
  generalized, type I*
  juvenile, type II*,
G^{m2} Gangliosidosis
  Type 1, Tay-Sachs disease*
  Type 2, Sandhoff disease*
  Type 3, juvenile
Krabbe disease*
Metachromatic Leucodystrophy*
Niemann–Pick disease*
Refsum disease
Wolman disease
Hyperlipoproteinemia, type II

Disorders of carbohydrate metabolism
Fucosidosis
Galactosemia*
Galactokinase deficiency
Glycogen storage disease, type II (Pompe)*
Glycogen storage disease, type III
Glycogen storage disease, type IV
Mannosidosis
Glucose-6-PO^4 dehydrogenase deficiency

Amino acid and related disorders
Argininosuccinic aciduria
Cystinosis
Citrullinemia (?)
Congenital hyperammonemia, type II
Hyperlysinemia (?)
Maple syrup urine disease
  severe infantile*
  intermittent
Methyl malonic aciduria
Homocystinuria
Cystathioninuria
Histidinemia

Mucopolysaccharidoses
MPS IH (Hurler)*
MPS IS (Scheie)
MPS II (Hunter)*
MPS III, A (Sanfilippo A)
MPS III, B (Sanfilippo B)
MPS IV (Morquio) (?)
MPS VI (Maroteaux–Lamy)
I-cell disease (?)

Miscellaneous
Acatalasemia
Adrenogenital syndrome*
Lesch–Nyhan syndrome*
Lysosomal acid phosphatase deficiency*
Xeroderma pigmentosum
Sickle-cell anemia
Myotonic muscular dystrophy (?)
Orotic aciduria (?)
β-thalassemia*
Anencephaly, spina bifida*

cessfully diagnosed in the early weeks of pregnancy. The near future should also see the development of an endoscope for viewing and photographing the embryo *in utero*.

The physician whose practice confronts him with cases requiring genetic counseling can hardly remain abreast of new developments in this field. He should therefore keep contact with a laboratory that specializes in prenatal diagnosis. If he then thinks that a particular case requires such tests, he can first check back with the laboratory to make sure that the indications suffice and that a diagnosis of the anomaly in question is possible. If and only if the laboratory confirms this should he then broach the matter with his patient.

Before going ahead with the test, patients must be informed about the possibilities and the dangers of the test methods. They should know that the first test may be unsuccessful and that the amniocentesis may have to be repeated. It must also be made quite clear that a negative test result does not guarantee a healthy child except for the one specific defect that has been excluded. The risk figures for other undetectable defects remain in force.

As a rule, the laboratory in question will explain all this in detail. The physician can, however, provide much-needed psychological support. It is he who will have to determine whether the couple in question would be willing to act upon a positive diagnosis or whether personal and/or religious convictions will preclude the interruption of an established pregnancy in any case. The implications of prenatal diagnosis make great demands on the people involved and there is little point in initiating such a procedure unless there is reason to think that it will truly help to bring a healthy child into the world.

10 Other Diseases Without a Simple Mode of Inheritance

Many diseases not commonly regarded as hereditary are heavily influenced by genetic factors. The knowledge of and about such a genetic liability within a family permits the general practitioner to direct his watchfulness, thus leading to an early diagnosis or, even better, preventive measures. Genetic counsel, in the stricter sense, will usually be required only if a family manifests an unusual number of similar diseases and if the circumstances indicate the existence of a Mendelian mode of inheritance.

The first question that arises is whether, in fact, the disease has a particular form that is subject to a simple mode of inheritance. For example, the careful pedigree analysis of a "cancer family" led Gardner and his associates to the discovery of the syndrome that now bears his name. The practically inevitable cancer of the intestine turned out to be a late development of an intestinal polyposis which, together with atheromata, fibromata, and osteomata, belongs to the pleiotropic picture of an autosomal dominant disease. Another autosomal dominant example is the already discussed malignant hereditary retinoblastoma (see p. 31). The occasional family with an unusual massing of cancer occurrence has also been reported. If the growths tend to occur at an early age and if different types of tumors develop in the same patient, then a possible genetic disposition with an autosomal-dominant mode of inheritance must be taken into consideration. In numerous families with multiple deaths due to myocardial infarction at an early age, the cause of the vascular complications could be traced to the hereditary, incomplete autosomal-dominant hypercholesterolemia (hyperlipoproteinemia, type 2).

If the possibility of a simple mode of inheritance has been eliminated, there remain two major groups of diseases: those with a high familial incidence, frequently raising the suspicion that *a single gene with exceedingly weak penetrance is the culprit,* and those where the *multifactorial system* alone provides anything approaching a reasonable explanation. Common to both groups is the fact that exogenous factors seem to play a considerable if not decisive role in the manifestation of the gene(s).

A good example of the former group is diabetes mellitus. Despite the fact that this disease is undoubtedly hereditary, the mode of inheritance remains unclarified. Every known mode of inheritance has been proposed and rejected. The major problem confronting a genetic analysis of diabetes mellitus is the lack of definitive diagnostic criteria, especially when it comes to distinguishing prediabetes from the normal condition. Clinically, the disease obviously presents a heterogenous picture. It is probable—though disputed—that genetic heterogeneity is at the root of the problem. But we do not know. The only thing that can be stated with certainty is that genetic factors are decisively involved in the etiology of diabetes and that the probability of developing diabetes increases in proportion to the number of diabetics among close relatives; but nowhere does the risk involved come close to the probability figures for the simple modes of inheritance. A case in point is the fact that not all the offspring of a marriage between two diabetics become diabetic as well, which would be the case were there a simple autosomal-recessive mode of inheritance at the root of the disease.

In counseling, the first step must be to make a precise diagnosis of the type of diabetes present and to identify or exclude special forms on the basis of clinical and biochemical data, personal history, and family anamnesis. In fact, each case deserves a detailed family analysis. Only on this basis can risk figures be calculated. Still, sufficiently large series are not available to give information on empiric risk figures for each special type and each single constellation.

The lack of diagnostic criteria for prediabetes and the heavily disputed question of genetic heterogeneity for diabetes mellitus is mirrored in the vast discrepancies between the various sets of data that are available for the calculation of the empiric risk. The most important single criterion to be considered is the age of onset in the index patient. The most recent available risk figures based on this differentiation alone may be the ones given by Darlow et al. (1973; see Table 10.1). If the risks for second- and third-degree relatives of an index patient are sought, the risk figures of the table should be about halved.

The data are derived empirically from a large sample collected in Scotland. They apply only to this population under

Table 10.1 Risk Figures for First-Degree Relatives of
Patients with Diabetes Mellitus by
Age of Onset

	Risk of diabetes by age (%)			
	25	45	65	85
Population	0.2–0.3	0.5–0.9	1.7–3.8	1.4–9.2
Proband onset				
Under 25	8	13	17	25
Over 25	(1)	(2)	9	21

Data from Darlow *et al.* (1973).

Table 10.2 Increased Risk for Clinical Diabetes in
First-Degree Relatives of Diabetics
as Compared to the General Population

Age of onset of diabetes in proband	Increased risk of clinical diabetes over that in the general population		
	Siblings	Offspring	Parents
0–19 years	10–14 ×	18–41 ×	2–3 ×
20–39 years	4–5 ×	6–13 ×	2–3 ×
Over 40 years	2–4 ×	1–3 ×	2–3 ×

Data from Simpson (1968).

the given circumstances. More generally applicable may be data that take into consideration the incidence of diabetes in the particular age group of the general population. Simpson (1968) calculated from her data the risk figures given in Table 10.2. All figures presented should be taken only as a crude general estimate, and a careful search into the history of the family to be counseled should follow to unveil possible further facts that might call for adjustments. Further affected members in the family point to a higher risk, and application of a factor between 1.5 and 4 was found appropriate depending on the age of onset and the degree of relationship of further affected relatives. Other factors to be considered are the severity of diabetes in the proband and the relatives, whether it is insulin dependent or not, and whether obesity runs in the family. One might thus arrive at a considerably higher or lower estimate than the general figures suggest.

The most important family factor in counseling a prospective diabetic parent will be a diabetes-positive or negative history of the spouse and his or her relatives, as well as information about the type of diabetes present in either family. If further affected relatives can be found in the family of both spouses, on theoretical grounds, in a multifactorial genetic disease such as diabetes, the risk should be considerably higher than in a case where the same number of affected relatives is known in the family of only one spouse. The higher genetic load may also reflect itself in an earlier onset and more severe manifestation. Empiric data in this regard are again missing, however.

The only certain facts are that the probability of the offspring of a diabetic manifesting the disease is considerably higher than average, and that the probability for the children of a marriage between diabetics is so high that such parents would be well advised to refrain from having children. Advisable, too, is a set limit to the number of proposed children in a union between a diabetic and a normal person, since social (the precarious health of the provider) as well as medical considerations (the hazards of pregnancy for the diabetic woman) are involved. Despite the fact that these are secondary consequences of the actual genetic disease, the advice would have to take into consideration the increased risk of malformation and of complications during the prenatal period for the children of diabetic mothers.

There is also a group of diseases that manifest themselves at a later date which show a definite though slight tendency to familial recurrence. Doubtless, the manifestation is decisively influenced by exogenous factors. To name a few examples, there are the cases of early atherosclerosis and myocardial infarction (apart from those caused by hypercholesterolemia and hypertriglyceridemia), rheumatic fever and the entire category of atopic diseases (asthma bronchiale, rhinitis vasomotorica, constitutional eczema of young children, and atopic dermatitis). With the exception of some extreme forms, very little is known about the specific genetic causes of the ocular anomalies of refraction.

In actual family counseling, a careful analysis of a particular case of this kind will often not produce anything really concrete in the way of facts and figures. All that can be said is that the children in a particularly affected kinship are subject to a higher degree of risk since the liability for the disease in question is especially pronounced. Should the prospective parent himself be affected, the risk is correspondingly higher. But, and this is an important but, apart from very special cases, there is rarely sufficient reason to oppose propagation altogether. *Objections became grave only when two people with the same disease wish to marry, and the disease is a severe one, not amenable to either preventive or therapeutic measures.* In other cases, genetic advice may actually help to ensure preventive measures, competent supervision, and early diagnosis and treatment for endangered children.

11 Oligophrenia and Mental Illness

In general, this category of illnesses involves the same principles that were developed in the preceding chapters in order to arrive at a genetic prognosis. Some forms of oligophrenia, for instance, follow a simple Mendelian mode of inheritance. Others can be traced to microscopically visible chromosome changes. There is also a category whose genetic roots are best explained in terms of a multifactorial genetic system. Despite this, the entire chapter will be devoted to these diagnoses, and for two very specific reasons:

1. *Oligophrenia and mental illness are frequent. Taken together, they include several percent of the entire world population.*
2. *For both counselor and counseled, problems in this category tend to involve a particularly complex mixture of genetic, psychological, and social considerations.*

The limitations of this book will not permit a detailed discussion. For further information, the reader is referred to Volume V, 2 of the *Human Genetics Handbook,* edited by P. E. Becker. In this volume, various authors discuss all the questions in this area for which genetic research has found some sort of an answer.

Oligophrenia Oligophrenia is not clearly distinguishable from what we describe as "normal intelligence." The borderline is vague and the transition is continuous. It comes as no surprise, therefore, to learn that the definition of the term is hotly disputed. In general, however, scientists agree that the line between "physiological stupidity" and a light case of oligophrenia can be drawn at an IQ of about 70. Taking this figure as the starting point, the estimated frequency of individuals with an IQ lower than 70 is, in various populations, somewhere between 1 and 3% (for detailed figures, see Zerbin-Ruedin (1967).

There are many different exogenous and genetic causes for oligophrenia; seen as a whole, though, the cases fall into two relatively definite categories (Table 11.1): one, a more numerous high-grade group and two, a less numerous low-grade group. The dividing line between the two groups falls at an IQ of about 50. Patients with an IQ of 70 to 50, the group of high-grade mental defectives, are usually described as "feeble-minded" or "morons," whereas those with an IQ of less than 50 are classed as "imbecile" or—in the worst case—as "idiots."

From the genetic standpoint, the two groups are distinctly different. The composition of group 2 is particularly uneven. It is in this group that the majority of exogenous cases are to be found—i.e., these caused by birth defects, traumatic lesions of the brain, and cerebral diseases during infancy. Statistics consequently show that most of these cases are sporadic; i.e., the only cases in otherwise normal—relative to the average population—families. *Under no circumstances can it be assumed, however, that all severe cases of oligophrenia have an exogenous cause and that therefore the genetic risk in relation to further children is negligible.* Although this assumption is frequently correct, especially in those cases where a clinical examination proves exogenously induced brain damage, there are cases where it would be totally false; group 2 also includes the many forms of oligophrenia subject to a simple Mendelian mode of inheritance.

Most of these forms of oligophrenia belong to the autosomal-recessive mode. Since the Western family unit tends to be fairly small, it often happens that the patient is the only case in the entire kinship (see Chapter 5). Before any counseling can take place, the patient must be thoroughly examined in order to make sure that his is not a case of autosomal-recessive form of oligophrenia. For a survey of these hereditary forms, see Stanbury et al. (1970), Bickel and Cleve (1967), and G. Koch (1967). Another possibility to be considered is that of a dominant new mutation such as tuberous sclerosis.

Group 2 also includes the various autosomal and gonosomal chromosome aberrations already discussed in Chapter 7. There is also a special subgroup consisting of the survivors of fetal erythroblastosis as a consequence of Rh incompatibility.

Having eliminated the cases of definitely exogenous origin and those that are of clearly genetic origin, there remains a large number that defy explanation within the limits of our present knowledge. Where these cases are an isolated incident in an otherwise normal family, further propagation need not be discouraged. The opposite is true if there are more

Table 11.1 Simplified and Classified Survey of the Typical Characteristics of High- and Low-Grade Mental Defectives

	Degree of defect	
	Mild (Group 1) (high-grade)	Severe (Group 2) (low-grade)
IQ	About 57	About 17
Psychological classification	Simpleton, moron, feeble-minded, high-grade	Imbecile, idiot, low-grade
Predominant medical classification	Physiological, aclinical, uncomplicated, idiopathic, residual	Pathological, clinical
Incidence of group in population	Common: 2%	Uncommon: ¼%
Proportion of group in hospital	Few: 3%	Many: 25%
Sex incidence	Females predominate	Males predominate
Frequent additional symptoms	Psychological abnormalities, associated with behavior disorders	Associated with physical malformations, neurological abnormalities
Mental capacity in absence of disease	Subcultural, below average	Normal
Biological classification	Fertility usually normal or heightened	Nonfertile
Status of relatives	Parents, brothers and sisters rather frequently defective but not sharply distinguished from normals	Parents rarely defective; brothers and sisters occasionally defective and sharply distinguished from normals
Traditional views on causation	Primary, endogenous, hereditary, intrinsic	Environmental, secondary exogenous, extrinsic
Typical hereditary causes	Common genes; multiple additive genes; sex chromosome aberrations	Rare specific genes; autosomal aberrations
Typical environmental causes	Deprivation; cerebral disease or injury in childhood; antisocial environment	Prenatal maternal influences; cerebral disease or injury in very early life
Social and familial conditions	Very poor	Average
Physical measurements	Means and variabilities within normal range	Means below normal; increased variabilities
Treatment aims	Special education; socialization	Elementary training; nursing care

Data, slightly modified, from Penrose (1963; cited by Zerbin-Ruedin, 1967).

cases, especially within the closer degrees of kinship such as parents and siblings.

For the high-grade mental defectives (group 1) the pattern is entirely different from that of the heterogenous group of imbeciles and idiots. As a rule, there are far fewer cases of dramatic exogenous origin than with the severe group, even though exogenous causes do exist now and then. There is also relatively little in the way of marked neurological abnormalties or noticeable externals. Instead, there is a *distinct pattern of familial recurrence*. Whereas the patients in group 2 usually possess normal parents and only occasionally affected siblings, the percentage of affected relatives in group 1 is very high.

Empiric risk figures derived from research data for "idiopathic" cases—i.e.,—those cases where no plausible exogenous cause can be found—are about 25 to 35% for the mothers, somewhat less for the fathers, between 10 and 40% for siblings, and between 15 and 50% for direct descendants. Even for cousins, the figures are between 3 and 25%, and for nephews and nieces, between 3 and 24%. The figures vary sharply, primarily because there are no set criteria defining the various conditions. The data do, however, indicate unequivocally the strong influence of genetic factors. To make matters really difficult, families with definite cases of oligophrenia usually contain a number of borderline cases as well. Even in the cases where the high-grade deficiency has a plausible exogenous cause, a careful pedigree usually shows an above-average percentage of other cases of oligophrenia among close relatives.

The data referring to this group also do not correspond with any known simple mode of inheritance. Instead, the facts tend to correspond more closely to the hypothesized multifactorial system.

The familial frequency of high-grade mental deficiency is responsible for the usual side effect in these cases, namely, that the social level of family life is very poor. A feeble-minded mother will create a very unfavorable environment for her children and thus additionally inhibit their normal development. In such families, exogenous and genetic factors combine in a particularly detrimental situation. Limiting the progeny in such families would seem very desirable, given the above facts. Unfortunately, it is precisely this group of high-grade mental defectives and the borderline cases who are the least capable of exercising responsible control over their propagation.

Example 8: The twenty-four-year-old female patient complains of periodic panic states resembling claustrophobia that have been going on for years. According to her mother, these attacks are combined with severe unrest. Apart from this, the patient suffers from a severe "liability of the vegetative nervous system with circulatory disturbances." A medical case history gives no evidence of any special illness; however, the patient was placed in a school for retarded children shortly after her schooling began. When she left school at 15, she was still in fourth grade. Since then, for nine years, she has been working in a Jugendwerkheim (a youthwork home for people with limited mental capacity) under protected conditions. She can read simple things but can only write her name and is incapable of the most elementary mathematical calculation; she can handle money only on the most primitive of levels. Besides this, the patient is highly sexed and virtually uncontrollable; in connection with her claustrophobia, she has the inclination to roam the streets and meet "nice men."

Her father was a farm laborer, and, according to report, feebleminded as well. The mother's schooling terminated with fifth grade in elementary school. A sister has completed elementary school and has learned a trade. The family doctor and the mother applied for permission to sterilize the patient. The girl herself was persuaded to agree to this step. Two neurologists, appointed by the medical board, examined the patient and approved the sterilization. One opinion stated: "apart from the clear eugenic indication (oligophrenia of mother, daughter, and probably father as well) there is also a medical reason for the sterilization, since the patient would almost certainly experience a deterioration of her coordination problems and a worsening of her already severe panic states if she were to become pregnant."[1]

The above reasoning is obviously eugenic as well as medical. These mixed eugenic-medical or eugenic-social considerations tend to be almost the most important factors in decisions concerning oligophrenia and mental illness.

In this example, permission was granted and the sterilization took place.

Mental Illness   Here we will briefly discuss the various forms of schizophrenia and the manic-depressive psychoses. We cannot go into the many details for either of these categories at this point and refer the reader to Zerbin-Ruedin (1967) for the most recent collection of genetic data about this area [see also Rosenthal and Kety (1969)].

With schizophrenics it is particularly difficult to establish simple guidelines because both the definition of the disease and its causes are hotly disputed and we are confronted with a number of different hypotheses for both. On the one hand, most twin series show a comparatively higher concordance for monozygotic twins than for dizygotic twins, and close relatives of schizophrenic probands will manifest the anomaly

[1] We gratefully acknowledge the contribution of this case history by Dr. Vollbracht, Head of the Consultation Commission of the Berlin "Aerztekammer."

with a much higher degree of probability than the mean population. On the other hand, there is no proof that these factors are due solely to the genetic constitution of a family. The psychoanalytical school of psychiatry has argued convincingly that the psychological constellation within a family is a very important factor in deciding whether or not a child will later develop schizophrenia. Further support for this hypothesis resulted from research with a series of discordant monozygotic twins (Tienari, 1963).

Support for the genetic hypothesis, on the other hand, derives from the studies of Heston (1966), who followed children of schizophrenic women separated from their mothers within a few days following birth who had no further contact with their mothers and did not live with maternal relatives. This experimental group showed the same incidence of schizophrenia as expected from general data on offspring of schizophrenics. Five of 47 children were affected, whereas none of the 50 children of a matched control group became schizophrenic. Half of the remaining children of schizophrenic women displayed a significant excess of psychosocial disability; the other half were notably successful adults.

This problem, however important it may be for research into the causality and for therapy, is of secondary importance in family counseling. The practical aim here is to prevent the conception of children who will have a much higher than average chance of becoming mentally ill. Whether the increased probability is due to genetic causes or to a singularly unfortunate family situation—or, most probably, to both—is finally, in terms of the practical aim, immaterial. Here, as elsewhere in actual practice, empiric risk figures can be used. A summary of these in accordance with the figures of various authors is given in Table 11.2. The figures given in the table are only the starting point in our work. An actual case will, as usual, consist of particulars, and the doctor will attempt an exact prognosis based on these, the specific form of the disease, and the genetic circumstances within the family concerned.

The familial risk is higher for the nuclear group of schizophrenia (hebephrenia, catatonia) than for the peripheral group; it is higher among siblings having one or even both parents affected than where the parents are normal, etc.

We ourselves would tend to dissuade from propagation any patient who has himself suffered from a definitely diagnosed case of schizophrenia, even if only a single attack has occurred to date. Some specialists, however, disagree and do not consider a single attack to be of such grave significance.

The problem becomes more complicated when the siblings of schizophrenics wish to marry and have children. Advice in these cases will be very individual. It will necessitate a care-

Table 11.2 Survey of the Empiric Risk Figures for Schizophrenia and Schizoidia (Corrected Percentages) among Relatives of Schizophrenics[a]

	Research series by Kallmann, 1938, 1946				Empiric risk figures for schizophrenia according to numerous series			
	Schizophrenia	Schizoidia	Schizophrenia	Schizoidia	Luxenburger, 1939	Kallmann, 1946	Schulz, 1952	Sjøgren, 1957
Average	0.85	—	0.85	2.9	0.85	0.3–1.5	0.8	0.7–3.0
Spouses	—	—	2.1	3.1	—	—	—	~1.0
Siblings	11.5 (20.5)[b]	10.0	14.3	31.5	10.8	4.5–11.7 (20)[b]	8.0–10.0	7.0–15.0
Half-siblings	7.6[c]	—	7.0	12.5	—	—	—	—
Step-siblings	—	—	1.8	2.7	—	—	—	—
MT	81.7	—	85.8	20.7	—	68.3	—	—
DT	12.5	—	14.7	23.0	—	14.9	—	—
Children	16.4	32.6	16.4	32.6	16.4	8.3–9.7	14.0	7.0–16.0
Parents	10.3	—	9.2	34.8	—	7.1–9.3	5.0	5.0–10.0
Uncles, aunts	—	—	—	—	—	—	—	—
Cousins	—	—	—	—	1.8	2.6	1.3	2.0
Grandchildren	4.3[d]	23.0	4.3	22.8	3.0	—	—	3.0–4.0
Nephews, nieces	3.9[e]	6.2	3.9	6.8	1.8	1.4–3.9	1.7	3.0
Grandparents	1.5	—	—	—	—	—	1.0	—
Children with two schizophrenic parents	68.1	17.1	68.1	17.1	—	53.0	40.0	38.0–68.0

[a] Data from Kallman's publications and other surveys. Blanks indicate respective degree of kinship not covered by author in question (Zerbin-Ruedin, 1967).

[b] With one schizophrenic parent.

[c] 1.7% if descended from normal parent; 24.0% if descended from schizophrenic parent.

[d] 1.3% with two normal parents.

[e] 2.5% if both parents are normal. For ascertained cases the corresponding figures are 3.0 and 1.9.

ful evaluation of the various factors: other cases in the family, especially whether the parents are affected; the age of the proband; his entire way of life to date (failure in school and at work? "schizoid" tendencies? indications of neurosis?). The prognosis as well as the counsel should preferably result from a close collaboration between the family doctor, a psychiatrist, and a geneticist.

Like schizophrenia, the various forms of the *manic-depressive psychoses* have no commonly accepted definitions. Again, detailed particulars can be found in Zerbin-Ruedin (1967). Twin research series show relatively high, but by no means complete, concordance with MT; the empiric risk figures for the various degrees of kinship are given in Table 11.3 (Data from different authors, collected by Zerbin-Ruedin, 1967). Again, the considerable variation in the figures of different authors is remarkable. The discrepancies result from the lack of a definition allowing the exact diagnosis of the trait; this is the real problem in sifting the proband material and applying the varying criteria for a diagnosis of the relatives.

Advice in cases of this sort will have to be very particularized and requires intimate acquaintance with the specifics of the individual case. There is a relatively high incidence of unusual talent among manic-depressives, and patients often contribute a great deal to society, despite their psychoses. Much will depend on the patient's own judgment of his situation. Perhaps he believes that his gifts and unusual experiences, based on his "being different," more than compensate for the burden of his psychosis.

Table 11.3 Empiric Risk Figures for Relatives of Probands Suffering from Manic-Depressive Psychoses

Degree of kinship	Number of affected relatives, %	Remarks
Siblings	Between 2.7 and 23% Usually about 10%	The risk for the siblings is increased if one of the parents is affected
Half-siblings Parents	1.4 to 16.7% 3.4 to 23.4% Usually about 10%	Here we find the doubtful cases and those that are "hypersensitive"
Children	6.4 to 24.1% Usually about 10%	Very little material available
Grandchildren	1.9 to 3.3%	
Cousins	1.2%	
Uncles and aunts	4.2%	

Data from Zerbin-Ruedin (1967).

In confidential discussion, the doctor will not be able to confine himself to the patient's illness but will have to talk about the siblings and the patient's children as well. This tends to apply to the whole area of psychiatric disturbances. *Genetic family counseling can only be beneficial as a part of an all-inclusive therapy.* In such cases, the doctor cannot rely solely on analytic and textbook norms or classification schemes. He will have to treat every case individually in terms of its particular human elements. Only in this way can he give responsible and convincing genetic counsel.

12 The Genetic Prognosis for a Consanguinous Marriage

Since ancient times, ecclesiastic and secular authorities have prohibited consanguinous marriages. This stand seems not to have had a biologic reason. As far as we can tell, it was based on social necessity, for the formation of a society and a civilization is inconceivable without an incest taboo. Historical reasons would probably account for the extension of the incest taboo to other degrees of kinship. Various societies made exceptions; some even tolerated the incestuous marriage between brother and sister—for instance, in ancient Egypt, where this privilege was reserved for the pharaohs· Christian civilization, however, frowns on consanguinous marriages. A marriage between first cousins is regarded as undesirable and the Roman Catholic Church still requires that the couple obtain a special dispensation (usually granted nowadays). But the ecclesiastic laws are also based on other than biologic considerations. This becomes obvious when one realizes that the church also forbids marriages between "spiritual" relatives—i.e., god-father and god-child.

Marriages between first cousins have always been relatively rare in our society. With increased mobility, a rather homogeneous population, and the small size of the Western family unit, their percentage of the total marriages has declined to less than 0.3% and in urban areas to less than 0.1%. Other civilizations frequently regard first-cousin marriages as eminently desirable for economic and family reasons, among others. In Japan, Schull and Neel (1965) estimated the frequency of such marriages (Hiroshima and Nagasaki) at 6%, whereas in isolated island villages in Japan nearly 29% of all marriages were between first cousins. Estimates for Bedouin tribes are equally high. Even higher frequencies of consanguinous marriages occur among the various populations of southern India. Often uncle-niece marriages (marriage to the daughter of a sister) are actually favored.

In our civilization there is a widespread belief that the children of consanguinous marriages are particularly imperiled and are much more likely to suffer from malformations and genetic diseases. Popular opinion even has it that such children are likely to prove less intelligent than the norm. For this reason, cousins who wish to marry frequently consult a doctor in order to obtain a competent answer to their questions.

The nature of consanguinity consists of the fact that relatives, because they have common ancestors, possess a greater number of common genes than the average percentage of common genes in the general population. The size of this additional fund of common genes will depend upon the degree of the relationship (Table 12.1 and Fig. 8.3). Children of consanguinous marriages therefore have a higher chance of receiving the same alleles for a gene locus from both parents—i.e., of being homozygous.

As an example, let us take another look at the important and—because of the distribution frequency—easily calculable probability for phenylketonuria.

In a normal family, with no previous record of any anomalies, first cousins wish to marry. Taking our example, is the probability that their children will develop phenylketonuria increased? If the mutual grandfather was heterozygous for the phenylketonuria gene, then the probability that his grandchildren inherited the defective gene is $1/2 \times 1/2 = 1/4$. That both grandchildren have the *same* gene from the grandfather equals $1/4 \times 1/4 = 1/16$. The same figures apply if the

Table 12.1   Share of Common Genes by Reason of Common Ancestry

Degree of kinship	Share of common genes due to common ancestry
Monozygotic twins	1
Parents, children, siblings, dizygotic twins	1/2
Grandparents, grandchildren, uncles, aunts, nephews, nieces, half-siblings, "double first cousins"	1/4
First cousins	1/8
First cousins once removed	1/16
Second cousins	1/32
Third cousins	1/128

grandmother instead of the grandfather was heterozygous. The total probability that first cousins will possess the same rare gene on grounds of their common ancestry is 1/16 + 1/16 = 1/8.

For phenylketonuria with a frequency of 1 : 10,000, there is an estimated heterozygote frequency of 1 : 50 (rounded off to the nearest number). This figure represents the heterozygote probability for either grandparent. The probability, therefore, that first cousins will both be heterozygous because of their common genetic background equals 1/8 × 1/50 = 1/400 or 0.0025%. The remaining 7/8 chance that the gene locus for phenylketonuria is not among the common 1/8 genes must, of course, be calculated in terms of the chance that both are accidentally heterozygous (Chapter 5); i.e., 7/8 × 1/2500 = 7/20,000 or 0.00035%.

In this case, the sum total probability of heterozygosity for the phenylketonuria gene is (rounded off) 0.0025 + 0.00035 = 0.00285% for the couple. Should they actually be heterozygotes, then of course their children will be homozygous for the phenylketonuria gene with a 25% probability. Therefore, the expectancy of phenylketonuria children from first-cousin marriages in apparently normal families would be 1/4 of 0.00285 or 0.00071%, which means not 1 : 10,000 as it is in the mean population, but about 7 : 10,000.

These probability figures could have been calculated directly: Children from first-cousin marriages have a 1/16 chance of being homozygous for any gene because of their parents' common ancestry. The remaining 15/16 of the gene complement has the same chance of being accidentally homozygous as the mean population. With a gene frequency $q = 0.01$ and a homozygote frequency of $q^2 = 0.0001$ in the population, the sum total risk figure for every child being affected with phenylketonuria equals:

$$1/16q + 15/16q^2 = 0.000625 + 0.00009375 = 0.000718$$

(The rounding off of the figures in the earlier calculations is responsible for the slight discrepancy in the results.)

The 1/16 value in the last calculation corresponds to the inbreeding coefficient (F) for the marriage in question. The general formula for the frequency (R) of homozygously affected offspring of a consanguinous marriage is

$$R = (1 - F) q^2 + Fq$$

or, since

$$p + q = 1$$
$$q^2 + Fpq$$

The inbreeding coefficients (F) of the most common consanguinous marriage types are summarized in Fig 12.1.

The relationship between the frequency of descendants homozygous for a recessive gene from consanguinous marriages and those accidentally homozygous from arbitrary unions is dependent upon the frequency of the recessive gene, as the formula and the preceding calculation demonstrated. The formula for the relationship is

$$\frac{1/16q + 15/16q^2}{q^2} = \frac{1 + 15q}{16q}$$

Consequently, the lower the gene frequency, the higher the value. With extremely rare recessive hereditary diseases,

FIGURE 12.1 Most frequent combinations in consanguinous marriages and the inbreeding coefficient.

Symbol	Description	Inbreeding coefficient
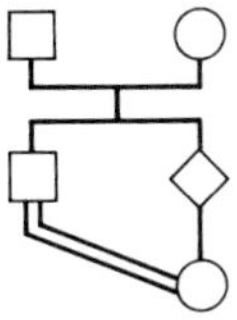	Uncle-niece marriage	1/8
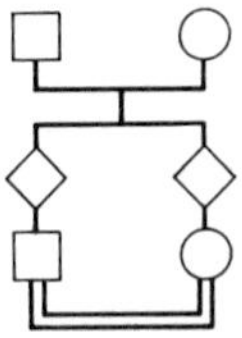	First cousins	1/16
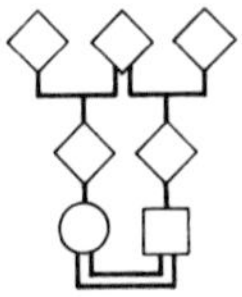	First-degree step cousins	1/32
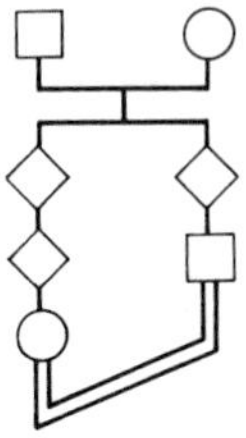	First cousin once removed	1/32
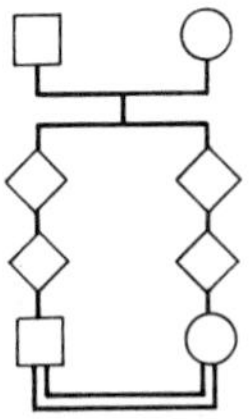	Second cousins	1/64

the probability is comparatively higher than with frequent recessive diseases.

As Table 12.1 shows, the increased probability for defective children dependent upon the common gene pool of the spouses diminishes rapidly the more remote the degree of relationship. *The marriage of a couple with a more remote degree of relationship than that of first cousins becomes unimportant from the point of view of family counseling.* Even if one partner were an established heterozygote, the probability of his second cousin being heterozygous for the same gene (on grounds of common ancestry) is only 1/32. The probability of a homozygous and defective child is therefore 1/128—i.e., less than 1%.

Let us return to the most frequent problem in practical counseling: the marriage between first cousins. The simplest case, for us, is when there is definite evidence that one partner possesses a specific gene. The probability that his or her cousin has inherited the same gene is 1/8 and the probability of homozygosity for every child equals 1/32. Should the potential disease or defect be a major one, this risk is considerable. Should both partners show slight evidence of an anomaly, an urgent warning would be in order. We would have to consider the probability that the cousins would both be heterozygous for the anomaly and that therefore their children would manifest an infinitely more severe case of the anomaly, since there is a 1/4 probability that they will be homozygous.

If nothing genetic that permits genotype identification is known about either cousin but a genetic anomaly with a simple mode of inheritance has occurred in the family, then one can calculate the probability of gene possession for each partner separately, according to the modes of inheritance discussed earlier. In a case of a marriage between normal cousins from a clinically normal family, the following considerations are important.

The above example of phenylketonuria probability shows an increase of 1 : 10,000 to 7 : 10,000. This does not seem a terribly serious increase. The trouble is that the calculation gives the figures for only *one* gene or allele; i.e., the one governing phenylketonuria or the relevant enzyme defect. The same calculation would have to be made in relation to every other gene locus in the human being, and we already know about 950 autosomal-recessive—mostly pathological—traits. An exact general formula establishing the general risk does not exist since the gene frequency of many of these anomalies remains unknown. Even more important, the degree of severity varies widely from defect to defect.

The number of genes in the human being is unknown. Educated estimates range between a minimum of 50,000 to 100,000 and a maximum of 6 to 7 million genes. As far as structural genes are concerned, the lower figures might be closer to reality. Furthermore, we must assume that each human being carries a number of genes that, in a homozygous state, would manifest themselves as hereditary defects. As a rule, then, an increased homozygosity in the population is undesirable. Moreover, it is reasonable to assume that in a number of multifactorial genetic systems, homozygosity considerably increases the probability of manifest illness.

Much research has been devoted to directly establishing the consequences of a common genetic load on the basis of first-cousin marriages. The results of these series are singularly unreliable. The problems are these:

1. The slight degree of the expected effects. Research would have to include very large series in order to obtain significant results.
2. The degree of the ascertainment bias occurring as a result of the above difficulty.
3. The difficulty in selecting a really representative control group.

The fewer the consanguinous matings in the population, the more such unions will represent special cases of geographic, socioeconomic, and psychological reasons for marriage, and the more the social status of the family will deviate from the population average.

A particularly well-planned and selected series of children from first-cousin marriages is the one examined by Schull and Neel (1965) in Japan. The frequency of consanguinous marriages in this society, plus the lack of discrimination against such unions, permitted the assumption that such marriages were relatively normal and not special cases, as they are in other societies. The children were examined at birth and again after 6 to 12 years. On the basis of an average age of 10, the results, in brief, showed a 3% increased mortality rate and a 1.6% increase in the probabiilty of such children developing a serious illness. Apart from this, children from first-cousin marriages were, on average, 1.6 cm smaller and weighed 0.3 kg less than their normal counterparts. Their IQ was 6 points lower and their grades in school (on a 1 to 5 scale) were about 0.1 worse. However, the series of first-cousin marriages showed a tendency toward a below-average socioeconomic status. Schull and Neel estimated that 12 to 35% of the recorded effect is due solely to these exogenous factors. Malformations are only slightly increased (Table 12.2). It is obvious that an estimate of the quantitative purely genetic disadvantages of a first-cousin marriage is incredibly difficult.

A possible advantage of a consanguinous match is the decreased probability, on grounds of the common gene complement of the parents, of biological incompatibility (e.g.,

Table 12.2 Distribution of Children with Severe Congenital Anomalies by City of Origin and Parents' Degree of Consanguinity[a]

(n = number of examined children; m = number of anomalies)

City		First-cousin marriages	First-cousin once removed marriages	Marriage of 2nd degree cousins	Parents unrelated	Total
Hiroshima	n	936	313	384	26012	27645
	m	17	2	4	293	316
	p	0.0182	0.0064	0.014	0.0113	0.0114
Kure	n	318	113	140	7544	8115
	m	4	2	1	58	65
	p	0.0126	0.0177	0.0071	0.0077	0.0080
Nagasaki	n	1592	412	637	30240	32881
	m	27	4	8	300	339
	p	0.0170	0.0097	0.0126	0.0099	0.0103
Total	n	2846	838	1161	63796	68641
	m	48	8	13	651	720
	p	0.0169	0.0095	0.0112	0.0102	0.0105

Analysis[b]

	χ^2	DF	p
Cities	7.269	2	$0.02 < p < 0.05$
Consanguinous marriages vs. normal marriages	11.775	3	$0.001 < p < 0.01$
Interaction	2.535	6	$0.75 < p < 0.90$

[a] Data from Schull (1958).

[b] Roy and Kastenbaum's method (1956) is used; see Schull (1958). There is a weakly significant difference between consanguinous and normal marriages.

the ABO or Rh factor in the blood group system) between mother and child. This advantage, though, quantitatively speaking, would be virtually insignificant.

In practical counseling, the most important factor in a case of a proposed consanguinous marriage is the careful search for indications of a genetic liability that would require the calculation of a particular probability. Apart from this possibility, one need only refer to the general, very slightly increased, genetic risk for the children of first-cousin marriages. There is not sufficient cause to discourage such marriages as a matter of principle.

Now and then, the question of the significance of a consanguinous marriage in the pedigree of someone's fiancé(e) arises. If the couple in question is unrelated, then consanguinous marriages in preceding generations are immaterial to the genetic load of prospective children.

If the engaged couple should be related as well, then the fact of a further consanguinous marriage in the common genealogy would increase—but only slightly—the calculable homozygosity probability for prospective children. No probability increase will have taken place in relation to autosomal-recessive diseases. Homozygosity of the respective gene would already have manifested itself in the offspring of the original marriage. Thus, the normal phenotype excludes this possibility.

13 Exposure to Mutagenic Noxes

The population of the Western world is exposed to an ever-increasing number of mutagens in its environment. The question about the genetic risk for the children of persons who have been inordinately exposed to such mutagens is being asked more and more often. To give specific advice about the dangers of a particular mutagen is not always possible on the basis of direct observational data in man. However, the results of experimental mutation research with mammals give us additional evidence of the effects of particular mutagens (Hollaender, 1971; Vogel et al., 1969; Vogel and Röhrborn, 1970).

Two types of environmental mutagens must be considered here: ionizing radiation, especially X rays, and chemical mutagens. The questions to be asked in relation to every possible mutagen are these:

1. How high is the dosage to which the germ cell is exposed?
2. Which stage of germ cell development is most vulnerable?
3. What type of damage does the mutagen induce? What happens to the genetic material in the cell?
4. Is the damaged germ cell viable and likely to reach fertilization?
5. What are the likely effects on the phenotype of the offspring?

Given the differences in spermatogenesis and oogenesis, these questions must be answered separately for the two sexes.

Radiation Exposure A comparatively low dose of ionizing radiation (100 R) will destroy a large part of the spermatogonia in the male mammal. This results in a more or less extended period of sterility. After a time, a repopulation of the seminal epithelium is effected by surviving A-spermatogonia, and the individual again becomes fertile. The majority of severe chromosome aberrations occurring in offspring derive from the presterile phase; i.e., they are the result of postmeiotic damage to the male germ cell.

An extrapolation of these results with animals to the human male indicates a *high level of risk if fertilization occurs within the first few weeks after radiation exposure.* The risk involves the possible transmission of structural (an perhaps numerical) chromosome aberrations. Germ cells with these anomalies can achieve fertilization. However, if we judge the behavior of induced chromosome aberrations to be similar to that of spontaneous ones, we must conclude that most zygotes so constituted will prove lethal at an early stage. Nonetheless, a considerable minority will survive, and the resulting children will suffer from malformation syndromes. It is therefore advisable to avoid impregnation within the first few weeks after the male germ cells have been exposed to acute radiation.

What are the chances of genetic anomalies if a longer period of time has elapsed between radiation exposure and fertilization? Mammalian experiments allow us to draw the following conclusions:

1. Radiation damages the spermatogonia. This means that damaged germ cells could occur for a very long time, perhaps a lifetime.
2. Radiation also induces recessive and dominant point mutations quite apart from the gross chromosomal damage. Germ cells with severe structural anomalies have very little chance of surviving the meiotic divisions. Point mutations and also some chromosome aberrations, on the other hand, can be transmitted to the subsequent generation (F_1).

To summarize, the risk of miscarriages and chromosomal malformation syndromes is slightly increased for F_1 if fertilization occurs after a longer time lapse; the risk is less than after postmeiotic radiation exposure. Syndromes due to dominant point mutations (see Chapter 4) are extremely rare. The increase in recessive mutations will not be manifest in F_1. Given these facts, a categorical warning against children seems excessive. Such a warning would require an unfortunate massing of negative circumstances in the individual case.

With women, the situation is somewhat different. If we extrapolate the results from experiments with mice, we must suppose that the mature oocyte (about the time of fertilization) is particularly vulnerable to radiation. In the early pronucleus stage, i.e., in the first hours after fertilization, there is a frequent occurrence of aneuploidies, especially monosomies. Most of these aberrations are lethal and will miscarry; a small number, however, may survive and show malformation syndromes. An increase of aneuploidies due to the radiation exposure of oocytes has been observed in experiments even outside the period when they are ripe for fertilization. Radiation also induces recessive point mutations in oocytes. The mutation rate is the same order of magnitude as that applying to spermatogonia exposure. These experimental results with mice should be valid for human beings as well.

The effect of the dosage rate is also important. A dose of radiation that is given over a longer period of time at a lower rate induces only $1/4$ the number of recessive point mutations in oocytes and spermatogonia as the same dose given all at once (possibly due to the action of repair enzymes). For genetic counseling, this fact suggests that extended exposure at a low dose rate is considerably less dangerous to human beings than a brief exposure with a high dose rate. However, such a dose/rate effect could not be observed for the post-meiotic stages of spermatogenesis.

The question that is very difficult to answer is this: *Which absolute radiation dose is to be considered dangerous?* In principle the rule holds that, genetically speaking, there is no such thing as a safe dose or a threshold effect. The doubling dose for mice could perhaps serve as a frame of reference. A doubling dose is the intensity of radiation necessary to double the normal spontaneous mutation rate in spermatogonia (Lüning and Searle, 1971):

1. Dominant morphological mutations (including skeletal anomalies): 16–26 R
2. Recessive mutations in 7 specific loci: 32 R
3. Autosomal-recessive lethals: 51 R
4. Effects due to structural chromosome aberrations (semi-sterility): 31 R

The above figures represent the doubling dose for acute irradiation of premeiotic germ-cell stages. With chronic exposure, the doubling dose is considerably higher. Genetically such treatment would be less dangerous. On the other hand, the doubling dose decreases in terms of the effects on postmeiotic germ-cell stages.

Example 9: The right testis of a 29-year-old man was surgically removed because of a seminoma. In addition, telecobalt therapy was given. For the following three years no signs of metastasis occurred. Hormonal contraception was used by the wife for the first two years thereafter and then discontinued because the results of an examination of the seminal fluid rendered a conception very unlikely. One year later, however, pregnancy was diagnosed. Both partners were greatly disturbed for fear of damage to the health of the fetus due to preceding radiotherapy.

Correspondence with the hospitals and the physicians of the patient resulted in an estimate of 150 rad for effective doses to the scrotal skin overlaying the remaining testis. The exact gonadal dose could not be determined; it could, however, safely be assumed to be below 150 rad. Since the radiation therapy did not affect the fetus but the paternal gametes, the mutagenic and not the potential teratogenic effect of ionizing radiation was to be considered.

For actual counseling, the long-range eugenic effects of radiation to the population are of no importance; our only concern is the immediate influence to the health of the expected child. According to the data discussed above, the therapy might have resulted in a fourfold incerase of the mutation rate had conception taken place shortly after exposure. Although the danger of chromosomal aberrations cannot be determined exactly, it can be assumed to be low. Most resulting aberrations will not be compatible with formation of functional gametes or with fetal development. The majority of mutations will be of the recessive type and therefore not affect the phenotype in the first generation. In later generations such mutations show up only if by accident or consanguinous marriage two identical alleles meet. Of concern would be dominant mutations, visible within the first-generation offspring.

Mutation rates of the few diseases transmitted in dominant fashion, for which estimates have been possible, were found to be about 1:100,000. A doubling of the mutation rate would increase the risk of such mutations to 2:100,000 for these gene loci. It must be considered, however, that so far in man about 1200 dominantly transmitted traits are known, half of them probably of major disadvantageous effect.

In addition, in the special case under consideration, according to extensive experimental experience one can expect that after three years' time most of the induced mutations will be eliminated or repaired. The actual danger for the expected child to show any clinically recognizable damage due to the previous radiation to the paternal gonads should theoretically be somewhat increased, but also for theoretical reasons this increase should be very small. It cannot yet be substantiated in experimental and epidemiological studies. From the viewpoint of genetics, therefore, there is no reason for major concern about the health of the expected child, nor would a warning for future pregnancies be warranted. Another matter to be taken into consideration for general counseling of the couple would, of course, be the individual prognosis of the patient and the problems deriving therefrom for the marriage and the family.

Chemical Mutagenesis
The effects of chemical mutagens are less easy to generalize about than those of ionizing radiation. For one thing, the mutagenic effectiveness of chemicals tends to be much more phase specific. For another, different groups of chemicals vary considerably as to the germ-cell stage they affect and as to the

type of damage they do. Though no general rule can be formulated, some germ-cell stages seem to be sensitive to all mutagenic noxes: the postmeiotic stages of spermatogenesis, the oogonia stage (only during embryonic development up to shortly after birth), and the oocyte stage of oogenesis around the time of fertilization. Cytostatica and antimetabolites are potentially mutagenic in normal therapeutic doses.[1]

The possible genetic damage due to hallucinogenic drugs —for example, LSD—has been discussed frequently. Experimental evidence, however, is still conflicting. The whole field of chemical mutagenesis is now developing rapidly. If a patient is treated with a high dose of an unusual or potentially dangerous drug, the doctor is on the safe side if he recommends the use of contraceptives during and about 8 weeks after treatment. In case the treatment has to be continued over a long time and the couple urgently wishes a child, he should seek advice from a specialist.

14 Teratogenic Effects During Early Pregnancy

The same group of compounds, which are known as potent mutagens—namely, cytostatics and antimetabolites—are also potentially teratogenic and should not be used, if at all avoidable, to treat illnesses during the first 3 to 4 months of a pregnancy. The most dangerous known chemical teratogen for an embryo, thalidomide, is no longer used therapeutically. A warning is therefore redundant.

Questions concerning the teratogenic effects of infectious diseases during pregnancy also arise. We will discuss this problem briefly, although neither it nor that of teratogenic drugs properly belongs to the field of genetic counseling.

Since Gregg's report in 1941, it is well known that rubella (German measles) contracted in early pregnancy will lead to a damaging infection of the fetus in a high proportion of cases. Prospective studies have demonstrated that these effects are highly dependent on the stage of the pregnancy during which the disease occurs. Even an unapparent illness of the mother may severely damage the fetus. The figures of Tables 14.1 and 14.2 can be used as a rough guide to estimate the risk. The data are, however, subject to many restrictions and difficulties of interpretation. Moreover, newer research data have shown that in addition to the classic rubella syndrome, further symptoms may be associated with intaruterine rubella infection. These include hepatosplenomegaly, hepatitis, jaundice, thrombocytopenic purpura, interstitial pneumonia, myocarditis, glaucoma, and anomalies of calcification of long bones. These effects may be associated with rubella infection during the second trimester. Hence, potential damage to the fetus is not restricted to rubella infection during the first trimester (Groscurth et al., 1973).

The correct diagnosis of an exanthematous disease in a pregnant woman is frequently a major problem unless general epidemiological data are clear-cut. During the acute phase of the illness, viruses can be found directly in blood or in nasopharyngeal washings. A positive result may be available within a week, but unfortunately, a negative result takes longer and is never really certain.

If a positive diagnosis has been made and an interruption of the pregnancy is out of the question, an intramuscular injection of 20 ml hyperimmune rubella globuline has been advocated. To date, results have been encouraging, but as yet a definite reduction of the risk has not been demonstrated. The vaccination of girls and young women may solve the problem. However, pregnant women should not be vaccinated; the same holds for women of childbearing age unless the possibility of pregnancy can be excluded at the time of the vaccination and for two months after.

Apart from rubella, only the virus causing *cytomegalic inclusion disease* has been proved to cause fetal malformation and infection. However, this disease is rarely recognized in the prospective mother, and since the symptoms are few and slight, no relationship between the time of infection and

Table 14.1 Anomalies in Live-born Children after Rubella Infection in Pregnancy

	Fetal age at time of maternal disease			
	1–4 weeks	5–8 weeks	9–12 weeks	1–8 weeks (incl.)
Anomalous/total number	14/23	19/72	10/127	39/104
Children with anomalies %	60.9	26.4	7.9	37.5

Data from Sallomi (1966).

Table 14.2 Incidence of Anomalies of Various Organs of 57 Fetuses Studied after Therapeutic Abortion Because of Maternal Rubella

Fetal age at time of maternal rubella	n	Anomalies %	% anomalies of			
			Lens	Heart	Inner ear	Skeletal muscles
0– 4 weeks	20	80	35	65	12	25
4– 8 weeks	31	58	48	45	13	16
8–11 weeks	6	(4/6)	(4/6)	(3/6)	0	0
0–11 weeks	57	68	45	53	11	18

Data from Töndury and Smith (1966).

fetal risk has yet been established. Various other viruses are held to be responsible for fetal malformations—e.g., the measles virus, influenza and hepatitis viruses, smallpox, and others. No definite proof has been established, however, and no risk figures are available.

15 The Human Element

Genetic counseling involves human beings as individuals. The most careful and accurate genetic evaluation of data will not be helpful if the results and the advice are not clearly understood by the patients. It is therefore extremely important to explain a particular situation with regard to the personality, the education, and the individual requirements of the patients. Human beings cannot be reduced to scientific formulas and no amount of scientific fact will compensate for a lack of human contact.

Unless there are serious objections, the final counseling session should take place in the presence of the parties concerned, both wife and husband or the engaged couple. The manner in which the facts are to be presented will depend very much on the education and emotional disposition of the couple in question. Without oversimplifying to an irresponsible degree, the facts should be presented in as straightforward a manner as possible. Simple diagrams can be a considerable aid to comprehension.

The results of the counseling session must be kept on file. It is also advisable to summarize the salient points in writing and to give them to the couple concerned. So often, facts that seemed clear and comprehensible during an actual discussion are confused and erroneously reinterpreted the next day. It is good practice to arrange a second session in order to make sure that the advice has been grasped and also to give the couple the opportunity for asking additional questions.

Although the calculation of hereditary probability is in itself a purely scientific procedure, *the resulting counsel is a therapeutic measure with far-reaching consequences.* If the case permits straight reassurance the matter is simple enough, but if the advice is negative, it is still meant to be effective. It is designed to affect an individual's or couple's entire way of life. It may even cause a disorientation of the personality or perhaps drastically alter a particular relationship.

The information that one spouse is the carrier of the defective gene, for instance, can easily lead to a massive guilt complex. This is best countered by emphasizing the chance distribution of the genetic load. To do this tends to be necessary anyway, for in order to understand the advice, the couple must accept that the laws of chance alone are responsible for the gene content, as well as the gamete which is finally fertilized. There is no personal responsibility involved. No one has any choice about the genes that he (or she) inherits from his (or her) ancestors, just as a new mutation, provided we did not actively and knowingly increase the risk, is an accident. Every human being carries some defective genes, and there is no way of making sure that his or her partner is not accidentally heterozygous for the same allele. *The counselor must make every effort to banish all false guilt or responsibility considerations from the discussion. It must be made absolutely clear that the purpose—our common purpose—is simply to prevent the misery imposed on the individual as well as his family through the birth of defective children.*

Such counseling also has "eugenic" effects since it helps to reduce the number of the genetically affected in families and thus in the population at large. Eugenics, in the strict sense of the term, aims at the reduction of pathological gene frequency as a whole. As the example of Huntington's chorea shows, this can be a direct consequence (although it is not a primary aim) of genetic counseling. Sometimes, however, counseling has the exactly opposite effect. Let us suppose that a warning against a consanguineous marriage or some other heterozygous union has been heeded because of the grave autosomal recessive danger. In this case, we have reduced the potential number of homozygotes—not very desirable from the eugenic point of view, since every homozygote who is too ill to propagate eliminates two defective genes from the total population gene pool. If one prevents the combination of two pathological genes in a homozygote, then the selection pressure against this gene is reduced and it must multiply unless we also limit the number of children in marriages between heterozygotes and normals. This, given the vastly greater heterozygote as compared to homozygote frequency, would, from the standpoint of population genetics, effectively balance the scales.

As in all medical consultations, we are obliged to tell the truth, but personal factors relating to the proband may make it imperative not to insist on the whole truth. If a pregnancy is in progress, for instance, there is no point in worrying the prospective mother unduly. Quite frequently it is sufficient to emphasize the positive aspect—as, for instance, the 95% probability of a normal child instead of the 5% risk of a severe malformation. This procedure is also indicated when the results of the analysis do not force the counselor to advise strongly against all further propagation.

As a matter of experience, genetic counseling is mostly a pleasant task; a chance to allay anxiety, reduce fear, and reassure. Only occasionally is it necessary to warn urgently and to confront the couple seeking advice with a very difficult and painful decision.

Many geneticists believe that counseling consists of merely providing the relevant probability figures on which the inquirers may then base their decisions. That the parties involved must ultimately decide for themselves is self-evident; that the geneticist can disclaim all responsibility for influencing the decision is, in our opinion, not really justifiable. There is no such thing as being totally objective. The manner in which the facts are presented alone will influence the decision, and the presentation is unavoidably subjective. Apart from this, we do not believe that it is either right or desirable to evade a personal commitment when it is desired and might be of help· It is in the nature of the doctor–patient relationship that the doctor assumes at least some responsibility for the patient, influences his decisions, and therefore must answer for them as well. The extent to which the doctor exercises these functions will depend largely on the patient's personality and the circumstances. The patient's personal disposition, philosophy, and religious convictions must be considered as well as the scientific facts.

If a strong desire for children on the one hand is countered by an increased probability of a genetically ill or malformed child on the other, a compromise solution of one child only might be recommended—provided, of course, that the risk is not too high. Should the compromise solution prove acceptable, the couple could satisfy their desire while keeping the risk within reasonable limits.

It is now possible to determine the health of an embryo with respect to a number of hereditary diseases, and the list is rapidly expanding (see Chapter 9). Prenatal diagnosis is a new way of helping families. In cases where it is possible, the geneticist need no longer confine himself to risk figures; he can offer certain knowledge about a particular growing embryo. Prenatal diagnosis presents considerable ethical problems without offering any ready-made solutions. How severe must an expected defect be in order to justify counsel for an abortion? Should such counsel apply only to embryos definitely suffering from such a defect, or is it to include carriers as well? Up to what stage of the pregnancy is termination justifiable? To be sure, the final decision rests with the prospective parents, but the doctor would be evading his responsibilities if he left it at that. A "right" decision in such cases is totally relative and should be arrived at in a clear dialog between doctor and patient. There is nothing academic about such decisions; the people in question will have to live with them. Their doctor can help them arrive at the solution proper to their particular case.

All the same, prenatal diagnoses make it possible to help couples who otherwise would not risk having children of their own at all. If the couple are prepared to take the consequences of a positive diagnosis, these tests allow us to avoid the birth of severely affected children.

If one is going to recommend that a marriage remain childless, then one must be prepared to help with the problems of birth control as well, or to at least recommend a reputable gynecologist or family planning center. Often, patients will not inquire directly, and yet it is a good idea to bring up the subject anyway. Despite the widespread use of contraceptives, there are still many erroneous popular prejudices as to the safety and effectiveness of the various methods. Besides this, genetically dictated birth control demands a very high standard of effectiveness, since it is not merely a matter of limiting the number of children in the family.

The change of attitude within the Roman Catholic Church in recent years has made it easier for devout Catholics to use hormonal, chemical, or mechanical contraceptives. But there is still much uncertainty in this area, and it might be necessary to recommend consultation with the patient's priest or a priest who specializes in problems of this sort.

In nearly every case of a genetic indication for birth control, known contraceptive methods will suffice. These methods do, however, require the intelligent and conscientious cooperation of the patients. Apart from this, all known methods have disadvantages, either side effects or an uncertainty factor. The relevant literature should be carefully studied. Most of these disadvantages and side effects can be avoided by the surest contraceptive method—surgical sterilization. This method is also the most disputed one, legally and religiously. The advantage of this method lies in its certainty; it obviates the continual conscientious application that the other measures demand. The great disadvantage of this solution lies in its irreversibility, a potential problem in cases of vicarious sterilization (a marriage might dissolve and the spouse, sterilized for the partner's sake, cannot now change his/her mind).

The same problem arises if an autosomal-recessive disease is the reason for avoiding procreation. In this case, the danger is strictly limited to the present combination of two heterozygotes. Neither partner would need to fear affected

children in a new marriage to a person who is not heterozygous for the gene. If the couple are considering sterilization, it should be remembered that a vasectomy is physically
a much lighter operation than a tubal ligation. A vasectomy
does not require hospitalization, and the risk of postopera-
tive complications is very low indeed. There may, however,
be psychological complications.

Because the effects are absolute, and because the pros and
cons of this question can never be totally objective, since it
ultimately concerns human reality and not abstract fact, there
is no general "proper attitude." Sterilization does, however,
remain a reasonable solution for those carriers who con-
sciously and out of a sense of social and personal responsibility decide never to risk passing on their defect.

In special situations, heterologous artificial insemination
might provide an alternative to childlessness or adoption.
From a genetic point of view, all cases are eligible in which
the risk is restricted to the male partner or—as in autosomal-
recessive diseases—to the particular combination of two
heterozygous individuals. The general ethical and legal problems are the same as with other indications and the same
rules apply in regard to the selection of the donor. In addition, however, special tests should be made in order to
ensure that the donor is not also a heterozygous carrier by
chance.

References

Treatises on Human Genetics

Becker, P. E. (ed.) (1964). *Humangenetik*, Vol. II. Stuttgart: Thieme.
——— (1964). *Humangenetik*, Vol. III, 1. Stuttgart: Thieme.
——— (1964). *Humangenetik*, Vol. IV. Stuttgart: Thieme.
——— (1967). *Humangenetik*, Vol. V, 1 and 2. Stuttgart: Thieme.
——— (1972). *Humangenetik*, Vol. III, 2. Stuttgart: Thieme.

Fuhrmann, W. (1965). *Taschenbuch der Allgemeinen und Klinischen Humangenetik*. Stuttgart: Wissenschaftl. Verlagsges. m.b.H.

Hamerton, J. L. (1971). *Human Cytogenetics*, Vols. I, II. New York and London: Academic Press.

Handbuch der Allgemeinen Pathologie (1974). Band 9, Erbgefüge. Berlin-Heidelberg: Springer-Verlag.

Harris, H. and K. Hirshhorn (eds.) (1971–1975). *Advances in Human Genetics*, Vols. 1–5. New York-London: Plenum Publishing Company.

Hsia, D. Y.-Y. (1966). *Inborn Errors of Metabolism*. Part 1: Clinical aspects, 2nd Ed. Chicago: Year Book Medical Publishers.

——— (1968). *Human Developmental Genetics*. Chicago: Year Book Medical Publishers.

——— and T. Inouye (1966). *Inborn Errors of Metabolism*. Part 2: Laboratory methods. Chicago: Year Book Medical Publishers.

Jadassohn, J. (1966). *Handbuch der Haut- und Geschlechtskrankheiten, Ergänzungswerk*. 7. Band: *Vererbung von Hautkrankheiten* (Hrsg: H. A. Gottron u. U. W. Schnyder). Berlin-Heidelberg-New York: Springer-Verlag.

Knudson, A. G. (1965). *Genetics and Disease*. New York: McGraw-Hill.

Lejeune, J. (1965). *Les Chromosomes Humaines*. Paris: Gauthier Villard.

Li, C. C. (1961). *Human Genetics: Principles and Methods*. New York: McGraw-Hill.

McKusick, V. A. (1975). *Mendelian Inheritance in Man*. 4th ed. Baltimore: The Johns Hopkins Press.

——— (1964). *Human Genetics*. Englewood Cliffs, N. J.: Prentice-Hall.

Milunsky, A. (1973). *The Prenatal Diagnosis of Hereditary Disorders.* Springfield, Ill.: Charles C Thomas.

Nachtsheim, H. (1966). *Kampf den Erbkrankheiten.* Franz Decker Verlag Nachf.

Penrose, L. S. (1973). *Outline of Human Genetics,* 3rd Ed. London-Melbourne-Toronto: Heinemann.

Stanbury, J. B., J. B. Wyngaarden, and D. S. Fredrickson (1970). *The Metabolic Basis of Inherited Disease,* 3rd Ed. New York: McGraw-Hill.

Steinberg, A. G. (ed.) (1961–1974). *Progress in Medical Genetics,* Vols. I–X. New York and London: Grune and Stratton.

Stern, C. (1973). *Principles of Human Genetics,* 3rd Ed. San Francisco and London: W. H. Freeman.

Vogel, F. (1961). *Lehrbuch der Allgemeinen Humangenetik.* Berlin-Göttingen-Heidelberg: Springer-Verlag.

Waardenburg, P. J. (1963). *Genetics and Ophthalmology.* Vol. II: *Neuro-ophthalmological part.* Oxford: Blackwell Scientific Publ. Ltd.; Assen, NL: Royal Van Gorcum; Springfield, Ill.: Charles C Thomas.

———, A. Franceschetti, and D. Klein (1961). *Genetics and Ophthalmology,* Vol. I. Assen, NL: Royal Van Gorcum; Oxford: Blackwell Scientific Publ. Ltd.

Witkowski, R., and O. Prokop (1974). *Genetik Erblicher Syndrome und Mißbildungen. Wörterbuch für die Familienberatung.* Berlin: Akademie-Verlag.

Wittinghill, M. (1965). *Human Genetics and Its Foundations.* New York: Reinhold.

References Mentioned in the Text

Bhasin, M. K., W. Foerster, and W. Fuhrmann (1973). A cytogenetic study of recurrent abortion. *Humangenetik, 18:* 139.

Bickel, H., and H. Cleve (1967). *Metabolische Schwachsinnsformen.* Humangenetik, Band V/2, Stuttgart: Thieme, 206–322.

Carr, D. H. (1969). Genetic factors in pregnancy wastage. *Med. Clin. North Amer., 53:* 1039.

Carter, C. O. (1964). *The Genetics of Common Malformations.* Second Internat. Conf. Congenit. Malformations 1963. New York: International Medical Congress Ltd., p. 306.

——— (1965). The inheritance of common congenital malformations. *Progr. Med. Genetics, IV:* 59–84.

———, and K. A. Evans (1971). Spina bifida and anencephaly in greater London—a family study. Fourth Internat. Cong. Human Genetics, Paris.

———, and J. A. F. Roberts (1967). The risk of recurrence after two children with central-nervous-system malformations. *Lancet, I:* 306–308.

Chen, Y. C., and Wolley, P. V., Jr. (1971). Genetic studies on hypospadias in males. *J. Med. Genet., 8:* 153.

Court-Brown, W. M. (1967). *Human Population Cytogenetics.* Amsterdam: North Holland Publications.

Darlow, J. M., C. Smith, and L. J. P. Duncan (1973). A statistical and genetical study of diabetes. III. Empiric risks to relatives. *Ann. Hum. Genet. Lond., 37:* 157.

Davidson, R. G. (1970). Application of cell culture techniques to human genetics. *Modern Trends in Human Genetics* (A. E. H. Emery, ed.). London: Butterworth, pp. 143–180.

Degenhardt, K.-H. (1964). Mißbildungen des Köpfes und der Wirbelsäule. *Humangenetik* (P. E. Becker, ed.), Vol. II, S. 489 ff. Stuttgart: Thieme.

Dorfman, A. (ed.) (1972). *Antenatal Diagnosis*. Chicago: University of Chicago Press.

Emery, A. E. H. (1970). Antenatal diagnosis of genetic disease. *Modern Trends in Human Genetics* (A. E. H. Emery, ed.). London: Butterworth, pp. 267–296.

Fogh-Andersen, P. (1942). *Inheritance of Harelip and Cleft Palate*. Copenhagen: A. Busik.

———— (1964). Recent statistics of facial clefts, pregnancy, heredity, mortality. *Early Treatment of Cleft Lip and Palate*. Internat. Symp. Zürich, 1964. Hrsg. R. Hotz. S. 44–51. Bern-Stuttgart: Huber.

Ford, C. E., and H. M. Clegg (1969). Reciprocal translocations. *Brit. Med. Bull.*, 25: 110–114.

Fraser, F. C. (1955). Thoughts on the etiology of clefts of the palate and lip. *Acta Genet.*, 5: 358.

———— (1970). The genetics of cleft lip and cleft palate. *Amer. J. Hum. Gen.*, 22: 336–352.

Fuhrmann, W. (1961). Untersuchungen zur Ätiologie der angeborenen Angiokardiopathien. *Acta Genet.*, 11: 289–316.

———— (1962). Genetische und peristatische Ursachen angeborener Angiokardiopathien. *Ergebn. inn. Med. Kinderheilk*, 18: 47–115.

———— (1968a). Congenital heart disease in sibships ascertained by two affected siblings. *Humangenetik*, 6: 1–12.

———— (1968b). A family study in transposition of the great vessels and in tricuspid atresia. *Humangenetik*, 6: 148–157.

———— (1972a). Fehlbildungen des Herzens und der großen Gefäße. *Hdb. Humangenetik*, Vol. III, 2 (P. E. Becker, ed.). Stuttgart: Thieme, pp. 257–327.

———— (1972b). Befunde bei speziellen angeborenen Angiokardiopathien (I). *Hdb. Humangenetik*, Vol. III, 2 (P. E. Becker, ed.). Stuttgart. Thieme, pp. 328–344.

———— (1974). Genetische Aspekte des mißbildungsproblems. *Handbuch der Allgemeinen Pathologie*, Band 9, Erbgefüge. Berlin-Heidelberg-New York: Springer-Verlag, pp. 523–580.

————, W. Seeger, and R. Böhm (1971). Apparently monogenic inheritance of anencephaly and spina bifida in a kindred. *Humangenetik*, 13: 241.

————, A. Stahl, and T. M. Schroeder (1966). Das oro-facio-digitale syndrom. *Humangenetik*, 2: 133–164.

————, C. Steffens, G. Schwarz, and A. Wagner (1965). Dominant erbliche Brachydaktylie mit Gelenksaplasien. *Humangenetik*, 1: 337–353.

Grebe, H. (1964). Störungen der epiphysen- und Gelenkentwicklung. *Hdb. Humangenetik* II (P. E. Becker, ed.), Vol. II. Stuttgart: Thieme, pp. 233 ff.

Groscurth, P., G. S. Kistler, and G. Töndury (1973). Zum Problem der Röteln im zweiten Schwangerschaftsdrittel. *Dtsch. Med. Wschr.*, 98: 570–574.

Hadorn, E. (1961). *Developmental Genetics and Lethal Factors.* London: Methuen; New York: John Wiley.

Hamerton, I. L. (1968). Robertsonian translocations in man: Evidence for prezygotic selection. *Cytogenetics 7*: 260–276.

Hanhart, E., and A. Kälin (1972). Zur Vererbung und empirischen Erbprognose der Lippen-Kiefer-Gaumenspalten anhand von 326 Fällen aus 309 unausgelesenen Schweizer Familien. *J. Génêt. Hum., 20*: 93.

Heston, L. L. (1966). Psychiatric disorders in foster-home-reared children of schizophrenic mothers. *Brit. J. Psychiat., 112*: 819.

Hindse-Nielsen (1938). Spina biflda. Prognose und Erblichkeit. Eine klinische Studie. *ActaChir. Scand., 80*: 525.

Hollaender, A. (ed.) (1971). *Chemical Mutagens,* Vols.' 1, 2, 3. New York and London: Plenum Press.

Hsia, D. Y.-Y. (1969). The detection of heterozygous carriers. *Med. Clin. of North America, 53*: 857.

Idelberger, K. H. (1939). *Die Zwillingspathologie des Angeborenen Klumpfußes.* Stuttgart: Enke.

——— (1951). *Die Erbpathologie der Sogenannten Angeborenen Hüftverrenkung.* München: Urban und Schwarzenberg.

Isigkeit, E. (1927). Untersuchungen über die Heredität orthopädischer Letden. 1. Uber die Erblichkeit des angeborenen Klumpfußes. *Arch. Orthop. Chir., 25*: 535.

Jörgensen, G. (1972). Befunde bei speziellen Angiokardiapathien (II). *Hdb. Humangenetik,* (P. E. Becker, ed.) Vol. III, 2. Stuttgart: Thieme, pp. 345–475.

Koch, G. (1967). Sondertypen des Schwachsinns (Erbliche Syndrome mit Schwachsinn). *Hbd. Humangenetik* (P. E. Becker, ed.) Vol. V, 2. Stuttgart: Thieme, pp. 431–442.

Krone, H. A. (1961). *Die Bedeutung der Eibettstörungen für die Entstehung menschlicher Mißbildungen.* Stuttgart: G. Fischer.

Larson, S. L., and Titus, J. L. (1970). Chromosomes and abortions. *Mayo Clinic Proc., 45*: 60.

Lenz, W. (1961). Zur Genetik des Incontinentia pigmenti. *Ann. Paediat., 196*: 149–165.

——— (1964). Anomalien der Geschlechtschromosomen, Gonadendysgenesien, Intersexualität, Hypospadie, *Hdb. Humangenetik* (P. E. Becker, ed.) Vol. III, 1. Stuttgart: Thieme, p. 387.

——— (1967). Anomalien der Autosomen unter besonderer Berücksichtigung des Schwachsinns. *Hdb. Humangenetik* (P. E. Becker, ed.) Vol. V, 2. Stuttgart: Thieme, pp. 340–430.

Linneweh, F. (1964). Fortschritte in der Diagnostik heterozygoter Merkmalsträger bei erblichen Stoffwechselkrankheiten. *Mschr. Kinderheilk., 112*: 169–173.

Lüning, K. G., and A. G. Searle (1971). Estimates of the genetic risks from ionizing radiation. *Mutation Res., 12*: 291–304.

Mikkelsen, M. (1971a). Down's syndrome: Current stage of cytogenetic research. *Humangenetik, 12*: 1–28.

——— (1971b). Identification of G group anomalies in Down's syndrome by quinacrine dihydrochloride fluorescence staining. *Humangenetik, 12*: 67–73.

———, and J. Stene (1970). Genetic counselling in Down's syndrome. *Human Heredity, 20*: 457–464.

Passarge, E. (1972). Genetic heterogeneity and recurrence risk of congenital intestinal aganglionosis. *Birth Defects, The National Foundation, Orig. Art. Series VIII*, 2: 63.

Pawlowitzki, I. H. (1972). Frequency of chromosome abnormalities in abortions. *Humangenetik*, 16: 131.

Penrose, L. S. (1967). Genetics of anencephaly. *J. Ment. Defic. Res.*, 1: 4.

———— (1963). *The Biology of Mental Defects*, 3rd Ed. London: Sedgwick and Jackson.

Pfeiffer, R. (1967). *Karyotyp und Phänotyp der autosomalen Chromosomenaberrationen beim Menschen*. Stuttgart: G. Fischer.

Ratnoff, O. D., and B. Bennett (1973). The genetics of hereditary disorders of blood coagulation. *Science*, 179: 1291–1298.

Reed, T. E., and J. V. Neel (1959). Huntington' chorea in Michigan. 2. Selection and mutation. *Amer. J. Hum. Genet.*, 11: 107.

Roberts, J. A. F. (1964). Multifactorial inheritance and human disease. *Progress in Medical Genetics* (A. G. Steinberg and A. G. Bearn, eds.) Vol. III. New York: Grune and Stratton, pp. 179 ff.

Rosenthal, D., and S. S. Kety (eds.) (1969). *The Transmission of Schizophrenia*. New York: Pergamon Press.

Sallomi, S. J. (1966). Rubella in pregnancy. *Obst. and Gynec.*, 27: 252.

Schull, W. J. (1958). Empirical risks in consanguinous marriages: Sex ratio, malformation, and viability. *Amer. J. Hum. Gen.*, 10, 3: 294–343.

————, and J. V. Neel (1965). *The Effects of Inbreeding on Japanese Children*. New York: Harper and Row.

Schulze, C. (1964). Anomalien und Mißbildungen der Kiefer, Lippen-Kiefer-Gaumenspalten. *Hdb. Humangenetik* (P. E. Becker, ed.) Vol. II. Stuttgart: Thieme, pp. 440 ff.

Simpson, N. E. (1968). Diabetes in the families of diabetics. *Can. Med. Assoc. J.*, 98: 427.

Slater, E., and V. Cowie (1971). *The Genetics of Mental Disorders*. London and New York: Oxford University Press.

Sorensen, H. R. (1953). *Hypospadias. With Special Reference to Aetiology*. Copenhagen: E. Munksgaard.

Tienari, P. (1963). Psychiatric illness in identical twins. *Acta Psychiat. Scand.*, suppl. 171.

Töndury, G., and D. W. Smith (1966). Fetal rubella pathology. *J. Pediat.*, 68: 867.

Tünte, W., and W. Lenz (1967). Zur Häufigkeit und Mutationsrate des Apert-syndroms. *Humangenetik*, 4: 104–111.

Vogel, F. (1963). Mutations in man. Proc. of the XI Internat. Cong. of Genetics (The Hague, The Netherlands, September.)

———— (1967). Genetic prognoses in retinoblastoma. *Modern Trends in Ophthalmology*, 4: 34–42.

————, and H. Dorn (1964). Krankheiten der Haut und ihrer Anhanggebilde. *Hdb. Humangenetik* (P. E. Becker, ed.) Vol. IV. Stuttgart: Thieme, pp. 304–506.

————, and G. Röhrborn (eds.) (1970). *Chemical Mutagenesis in Mammals and Man*. Heidelberg and New York: Springer-Verlag.

————, G. Röhrborn, E. Schleiermacher, and T. M. Schroeder (1969). *Strahlengenetik der Säuger L. Fortsch. Allg. Klin. Humangenetik*. Stuttgart: Thieme.

Wynne-Davies, R. (1964). Family studies and the cause of congenital club foot. *J. Bone Jt. Surg., 46B*: 445.

———— (1970). A family study of neonatal and late diagnosis congenital dislocation of the hip. *J. Med. Genet., 7*: 315–324.

Zerbin-Rüdin, E. (1967a). Idiopathischer Schwachsinn. *Hdb. Humangenetik* (P. E. Becker, ed.) Vol. V, 2. Stuttgart: Thieme, pp. 158–205.

———— (1967b). Endogene Psychosen. *Hdb. Humangenetik* (P. E. Becker, ed.) Vol. 5, 2. Stuttgart: Thieme, pp. 446–577.

Zetterqvist, P. (1972). *A Clinical and Genetic Study of Congenital Heart Defects.* Publication from the Institute for Medical Genetics of the University of Uppsala, Sweden.

Zoethout, H. E., R. E. Bonham Carter, and C. O. Carter (1964). A family study of aortic stenosis. *J. Med. Genet., 1*: 2–9.

Index